Hot topics in adolescent health
A practical manual for working with young people

Hot topics in adolescent health

A practical manual for working with young people

Sarah Bekaert

Advanced Nurse Practitioner

Radcliffe Publishing
London • New York

Radcliffe Publishing Ltd
33-41 Dallington Street
London
EC1V 0BB
United Kingdom

www.radcliffepublishing.com

Electronic catalogue and worldwide online ordering facility.

British Library Cataloguing in Publication Data

A catalogue record for this book is available from the British Library.

ISBN-13: 978 184619 301 9

The paper used for the text pages of this book is FSC certified. FSC ® (The Forest Stewardship Council ®) is an international network to promote responsible management of the world's forests.

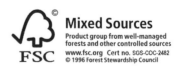

Mixed Sources
Product group from well-managed forests and other controlled sources
www.fsc.org Cert no. SGS-COC-2482
© 1996 Forest Stewardship Council

Typeset by KnowledgeWorks Global Ltd, Chennai, India
Cover design by COX Design Limited
Printed and bound by TJI Digital, Padstow, Cornwall, UK

Contents

About the author

Sarah Bekaert is an Advanced Nurse Practitioner for City and Hackney Young People's Services. Trained as a Children's Nurse at City University, she went on to gain a Masters in Sexual and Reproductive Health at Warwick University focusing on adolescent health care. She has published several books including Adolescents and Sex, Contraception and Sexual Health, and Women's Health. She is a member of the London Society of Family Planning Practitioners and is part of the Editorial Advisory Board for Children and Young People's Nursing: the journal for nurses caring for children and young people. She lives in Hackney with her husband and two daughters.

Dedicated to Charlotte Edith

Figures and diagrams

CD contents

Introduction

This book has been inspired by the work of the Hackney Teenage Health Demonstration Site 'CHYPS Plus'. Commissioned to pilot new and innovative ways of tackling adolescent health care, we set up a holistic health service to promote healthy lifestyles for young people. This involved building partnerships with a range of professionals to ensure ease of access to services which could improve a young person's health. Successful partnerships were numerous and included experts in the fields of dietetics, mental health, drugs and alcohol, fitness, education, careers and many others. Our most important partners of all were the young people of Hackney themselves.

In addition to setting up a hub to deliver these services, we also sought to take the model out to hard-to-reach groups, e.g. the Youth Offending Team, local colleges, Looked After Children, and others. Thirdly, we had a role in equipping other professionals working with young people to deliver health messages alongside their specific activity; for example, sports coaches and drama and dance groups.

It was through thinking about what would be the key health messages that we would like to get across to young people that I have brought together a body of knowledge to form this pack, which can then support professionals working with young people. It is designed to be dipped into according to sessions that are delivered to the young people within your organisation. The aim is to explain why the topic is important for young people, give some background information, make suggestions for activities to explore the subject with your group, and provide signposts to other sources of information on the subject.

Using interactive methods of delivery with suggestions for wider and varied resources, we cover an introduction to adolescence in Chapter 1: Puberty, and then explore the nitty-gritty issues that can affect young people in our society, e.g. body image, mental health, drugs and alcohol, relationships and sex (including contraception, sexual health, pregnancy and abortion). We also explore areas that lay down good foundations for health in later life such as healthy eating and exercise. In addition, there is a section on consent and confidentiality. (For those working with young people; this can be a tricky area as different professions have different codes of confidentiality) and child protection.

CHAPTER 1

Puberty

Remember Harry Enfield's character Kevin? The time when the delightful, chatty 12 year old turns into a disgruntled, grumpy teen? For those working with this age group, it can be difficult to accommodate the varying needs of a young person—each enters puberty at different times; each working through his or her relationship with a "new self" as well as relationships with peers, adults and family. In addition, the transition doesn't happen overnight and mood and communication can vary dramatically from minute to minute!

Puberty is the time when a child physically develops into an adult. For example, girls develop breasts and boys broaden out, and hair sprouts in all sorts of new places! Usually, puberty starts between the ages of 8–13 in girls and 10 15 in boys. Hence, in this age group there can be a wide range of shapes and sizes.

There are emotional changes too as a developing sense of self leads young people to a reshaping of relationships with peers, adults and family. The development of sexual feelings alongside the physical changes can cause embarrassment and confusion too.

This section will look at the physical changes that happen to boys and girls and offer advice on topics like body odour and acne to help boost self-esteem during this time. It will also look at the emotional changes that take place and how they influence social interaction.

Finally, we will look at areas where, as if puberty isn't complicated enough, other factors can make the journey even more complicated, e.g. disability, sexuality.

WHAT HAPPENS IN PUBERTY?

Draw two androgynous figures on large pieces of paper. Get the group to tell you about the changes that occur in puberty and draw these changes onto the picture.

According to the level of the group, bring out discussion on what might cause these changes, how they may happen at different times for different young people and the possible consequences of these changes.

BIOLOGY

Hormones

For boys, hormones travel through the blood and tell the testes, the two egg-shaped glands in the scrotum (the sac that hangs under the penis), to begin making testosterone and sperm. Testosterone is the hormone that causes most of the changes in a boy's body during puberty.

In girls, FSH (follicle stimulating hormone) and LH (luteinising hormone) target the ovaries, which contain eggs that have been there since birth. The hormones stimulate the ovaries to begin producing another hormone called oestrogen. Oestrogen, along with FSH and LH, causes a girl's body to mature and prepare her for pregnancy.

Boys and girls both begin to grow hair under their arms and their pubic areas (on and around the genitals). It starts out looking light and thin. Then, as they go through puberty, it becomes longer, thicker, heavier, curlier and darker. Eventually, boys also start to grow hair on their faces.

Growth spurt

Both boys and girls undergo a growth spurt during this time; some can grow up to four inches in one year. Naturally their appetite will reflect this; they need lots of food, ideally representing all food groups, in order to develop good bone strength, muscle and skin tone. The classic "teenager sleeping until midday", while annoying for parents, is a natural reflection of the sleep teenagers typically need for all this growth! (*See* Chapter 4 for more information on nutrition needs during this growth spurt.)

Changing shape

Boys' and girls' bodies fill out and change shape during puberty. A boy's shoulders grow wider and his body will become more muscular. There may be a bit of breast growth for boys; this is normal—it goes away for most by the end of puberty. In addition, boys' voices crack and eventually become deeper, their penises grow longer and wider and their testes get bigger.

Girls' bodies usually become curvier. Their hips get wider and their breasts develop. Sometimes one breast grows more quickly than the other, but most of the time they even out. Girls may start wearing bras around this time, especially if they are involved in sports or exercise classes.

Male reproductive organs

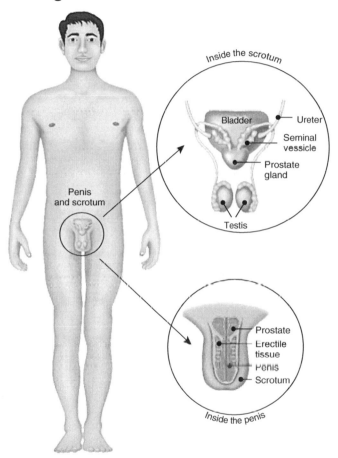

Figure 1.1 The male reproductive organs

The main function of the male reproductive organs is to make sperm and pass them to the female. The organs consist of two round glands called testes that lie in a special sac (scrotum) outside the body. Within the testes are tubules and ducts where sperm are produced. A duct, called the vas deferens, comes out of each testis and up into the pelvis. At this point, the seminal vesicle joins the vas deferens. The seminal vesicles add seminal fluid to the sperm. The duct then becomes the ejaculatory duct, which fuses with the urethra at the prostate gland. The duct is then called the prostatic urethra and carries both urine and semen through the penis. The penis is made up of vascular spaces and erectile tissue.

Female reproductive system

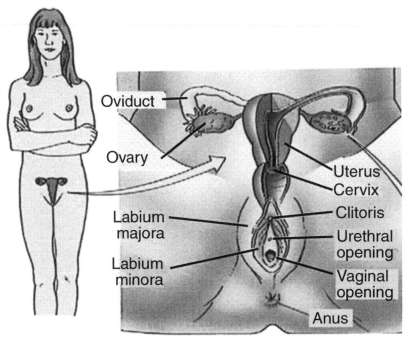

Figure 1.2 The female reproductive organs

The female reproductive system is designed to make eggs, to favour fertilisation and to house the growing foetus during pregnancy. The ovaries produce eggs (or ova) from follicles. The egg travels down the fallopian/uterine tubes to the uterus, where a fertilised egg will implant and the foetus develops. At the base of the uterus is the cervix, leading to the vagina where sperm can be introduced from the penis.

Fertilisation

Fertilisation takes place when a sperm and egg fuse. Once a month an egg is released from the ovaries (ovulation) and travels down the uterine tubes. If it meets sperm in the uterine tubes it may be fertilised. The fertilised egg then travels to the uterus and implants in the uterine wall, where the foetus develops.

Periods

Before contraception can be understood it is helpful to have an understanding of the menstrual cycle, as most hormonal contraceptive methods interrupt this cycle in some way. (*See* Chapter 9 for more information about contraception.)

The menstrual cycle is calculated from the first day of a period until the day before the next period starts. The length of the menstrual cycle varies for each individual and often from one period to the next. It can be as short as 21 days and as long as 40 days.

The menstrual cycle is controlled by hormones. The chemical messenger follicle stimulating hormone releasing factor (FSH-RF) is released by the hypothalamus, a gland in the brain. This hormone tells the pituitary, also in the brain, to secrete follicle stimulating hormone (FSH) and luteinising hormone (LH) into the bloodstream. These hormones cause the follicles in the ovaries to begin to mature.

The maturing follicles release the hormone oestrogen. Oestrogen causes the lining of the uterus to thicken. When the oestrogen level reaches a certain point it causes the hypothalamus to release luteinising hormone releasing factor (LH-RF), causing the pituitary to release a large amount of luteinising hormone (LH). This surge of LH triggers the most mature follicle to burst open and release an egg. This is called ovulation.

Inside the uterine tube, the egg is carried toward the uterus. Fertilisation occurs if sperm are present as the live egg reaches the uterus.

The follicle from which the egg burst becomes the corpus luteum (yellow body). As it heals, it produces the hormones oestrogen and, in larger amounts, progesterone, which is necessary for the maintenance of a pregnancy. Progesterone causes the surface of the uterine lining, the endometrium, to become covered with mucous, secreted from glands within the lining itself. If fertilisation and implantation do not occur, the arteries of the lining close off, stopping blood flow to the surface of the lining. The endometrium lining comes away as a period.

The drop in hormones from the ovaries stimulates the hypothalamus and pituitary gland to begin to release FSH and start the next cycle.

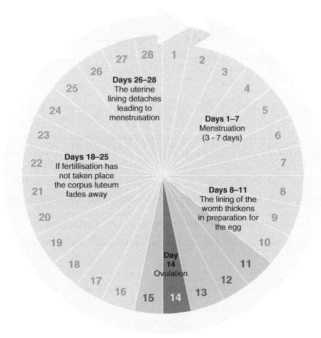

Figure 1.3 The menstrual cycle

THE CONSEQUENCES

Nocturnal ejaculation or 'wet dreams'

A wet dream is when a boy ejaculates semen in his sleep. It's normal, unavoidable, and totally natural. Apparently the average teenager has four erections every night and a wet dream about every three weeks. A boy may wake up remembering the dream or may sleep through it. It is more likely to happen at the weekend, as teenagers sleep longer and are more likely to dream!

Masturbation

Masturbation is the touching or stimulating of your own or someone else's genitals for sexual pleasure. Masturbation is a natural and normal way of exploring your own body. Naturally this is something that should be done in private.

Spots

Acne is a skin problem that usually begins in the young teenage years and can last until the early 20s or even later. It consists of mild to severe outbreaks of pimples and cysts. Cysts are lumps under the skin that have pus and other tissue in them, but do not come to a head like pimples do. These can sometimes cause scarring and blotchy, uneven skin colour. Unfortunately, acne hits people at a time when they most want to look their best. Acne can make teenagers feel embarrassed and bad about themselves. There are treatments that can help if acne is causing distress.

At the start of puberty, many hormones are released into the body. One of these hormones is androgen. Both boys and girls have androgen, but boys have more of it. Androgen affects oil glands in the skin of the face, neck, back, shoulders and chest. It makes the glands grow bigger and produce more oil (sebum). Bacteria on the skin make this oil thicken so that the pores become blocked, resulting in blackheads, pimples, and cysts. A teenager is more likely to get acne if one of his or her parents had it during adolescence. But even in the same family, some people may get worse acne than others. Girls tend to get it at a younger age than boys and it can worsen or 'break out' at certain times of a girl's menstrual cycle, such as just before a period. Boys often have more outbreaks than girls, and they often seem to get worse pimples and more cysts.

Ditching the zits

Self-help strategies

Suggestions for managing acne include:

- **washing**—Cleaning the skin can help, but even people with very clean skin can have problems with acne. Try washing the affected areas two to three times per day. Don't overdo it. Too much washing can cause other skin problems, such as dryness or skin irritations. Try to keep hair clean and off the face and neck, since oil from the hair can make acne worse
- **make-up**—Choose water-based, oil free products. Make-up worn during the day should be thoroughly removed at night
- **don't squeeze**—Do not pick or squeeze pimples. This can get germs into the skin around the pimple and make things a lot worse. It can lead to scarring of the skin too
- **avoid stress**—Stress can trigger an outbreak of pimples. Stress causes the release of chemicals into the brain that can make oil glands release more oil onto the skin. This is why pimples seem to magically appear on stressful days, such as at the time of an exam or special date
- **diet**—Many people think that chocolate cause pimples. Research has not been able to prove any such link, but some people find that it works this way for them. It is possible that a person eats chocolate when they are under a lot of stress, and that it is actually the stress that causes the pimples. However, healthy eating may help.

Acne treatment from your pharmacy

Some acne treatments can be bought over the counter at chemists or supermarkets. These treatments work by cleaning the skin and drying up excess oil. If you are using any form of treatment and your skin becomes very dry or irritated, stop using it straight away. It is a good idea to talk to the chemist before you buy a product to find out which treatments are the most useful.

Medical treatment

If the acne is bad, your doctor may prescribe medication or arrange a referral to a dermatologist. Medications can lead to huge improvements in how the skin looks and can reduce the number of new pimples. Medical treatment can include:

- antibiotics to kill the germs, which are part of the cause
- medications to reduce the amount of oil being produced
- medications to reduce the amount of androgen in the body.

Personal hygiene

During puberty the body goes through some very important changes, increasing the need for a regular regime for maintaining personal hygiene. Many teenagers and indeed parents find these changes embarrassing to discuss and many teenagers can be left in the dark about what they need to do to avoid embarrassment.

Body odour

Puberty causes the body to produce greater quantities of oils and sweat that can clog up the pores leading to spots, acne or sores. This coupled with increased activity can lead to foul-smelling and offensive body odour. This subject should be discussed in an informal and gentle manner so as not to make a big issue of it.

Boys should be told about the occurrence of wet dreams and the need for a morning shower, whilst girls should be educated on their menstrual cycle and how this can add to odours.

Parents or a trusted adult should discuss the variety of antiperspirant deodorants available and explain why they are needed; you can't simply spray deodorant as an alternative to washing. Clearly this temporarily masks odours but does not stop the problem.

What is the difference between antiperspirant and deodorant?

Antiperspirants contain aluminum chloride, or aluminum zirconium. These plug up the sweat glands and prevent sweating. Some people think this is a bad thing as aluminum is a neurotoxin, and it may not be a good idea to put it under armpits everyday.

Deodorant works differently; instead of plugging up the pores of sweat glands, it has antibacterial agents that inhibit the growth of the bacteria that cause underarm odour. Deodorant also won't stain some shirts like antiperspirants do. When sweat and aluminium zirconium mix, they can harm the dye in clothing and give yellow stains under the armpits.

Antiperspirant deodorant is basically an antiperspirant that also has a fragrance to get rid of odour.

The Internet has some very good guides on how to shave. YouTube is particularly good as it provides a visual demonstration. *See* 'How to shave like a pro' at www.youtube.com/watch?v=ALOKiXe1mSQ

Shaving (for men)

Step 1
Wet your face with warm water. You may want to hold a wet washcloth to your beard for a few minutes to soften the skin.

Step 2
Fill the sink basin halfway with water.

Step 3
Get out a new razor, or replace the used blade in your regular razor.

Step 4
Squirt a dollop of shaving cream into your hand or shake out shaving powder, then apply it to your beard in upward circular motions. The amount may vary depending on the thickness of your beard, but the area to be shaved should be covered uniformly.

Step 5
Shave downward, the way your whiskers grow, from your sideburns using long, even strokes. Apply light but firm pressure, pulling your skin taut before each stroke.

Step 6
Rinse your razor with warm water after every stroke or two to keep it from getting clogged with hair.

Step 7
Shave the area around your chin. Shave upward as necessary to make the area smooth. When shaving under your chin, pull the razor from your throat area toward your chin.

Step 8
Shave your upper lip, keeping the skin tight by curling your lip over your front teeth.

Step 9
Wash off any excess shaving cream and examine your face for straggling hairs. Check the edge of your jaw, around your ears, and near your lips and nostrils for missed hairs. Go back with the razor to shave any hairs you missed.

Step 10
Drain and wash out the basin and apply cold water or aftershave as desired.

Step 11
Moisturize. *See* www.ehow.com/how_2116_shave-face.html

Shaving (for women)

Shaving first became popular during World War II, when nylon stockings were in short supply and bare legs became a trend.

Here are some tips to ensure you cut down on the nicks and irritation that are so common to shaved skin.

1 Wet your skin and let it soften from the heat and moisture. You don't want to shave dry skin. Shaving is a natural exfoliator, and you'll clog up the razor with dead skin while putting yourself at risk for nicks.
2 Exfoliate your skin before shaving. It gets rid of all the dead skin cells that could clog up your razor, preventing a close shave.
3 Apply shaving foam.
4 Since your leg hairs grow down, you'll want to start at your ankles and shave up. For your underarms, you'll need to shave in every direction since the hair there grows every which way.
5 Be sure to change razors on a regular basis, as a dull blade can lead to nicks. Also, it's best not to borrow your guy's razor. His hair is coarser and will dull a blade.
6 When finished, apply oil or moisturizer. The skin on your legs has few oil glands and has a tendency for dryness.
7 Ingrown hairs are caused when the hairs curl back under the skin. Avoid them by exfoliating regularly and using body lotion.

Other hair removal techniques

Waxing–Waxing is the removal of body hair by forcibly pulling it out by the roots using some force of adhesion. This can either be done in a salon or home kits are available. The hairs stay away for longer than shaving.

Depilatory creams–Depilatory creams are good for short-term hair removal. They remove hair just below the skin's surface. Their disadvantage is that the chemicals that 'burn' off hair can also cause skin irritation. Those with very sensitive skin may not be able to tolerate depilatory creams.

For best results, first apply a warm washcloth to the area; this will soften the hair and open the follicles so the depilatory cream can be better absorbed. Never exceed the recommended time for leaving the cream on the skin. When removing the cream, use a washcloth to wipe it off instead of simply rinsing (additional pressure can help remove more of the hair shaft). This type of hair removal lasts several days.

Depilatory creams contain sodium thioglycolate and calcium thioglycolate to dissolve the keratin that makes up the hair. When these chemicals mix with the hair there's often a mildly unpleasant, sulphur-like odour that goes away when the cream is rinsed.

Test depilatory cream on your forearm before using it to determine whether your skin reacts to it adversely (some creams cause skin discoloration or staining; others provoke allergies). If your skin reacts when using a depilatory cream, wash the area with an antibacterial solution. You may need an antibiotic or cortisone cream to reduce the inflammation (see your doctor). Never apply a depilatory to an area that has any cuts, scratches or other wounds.

Laser treatment–Lasers produce a high-intensity ray of pure light, which gives off heat energy. This energy is absorbed by different body tissues, depending on the colour of the laser beam. That's why laser light can pass safely through the skin and destroy targeted cells under the surface without harming surrounding areas. For hair removal, the heat energy damages the cells at the root of the hair, thus preventing further growth. It probably won't remove all hair permanently, but should reduce growth significantly, and any regrowth is likely to be paler and weaker. Lasers are targeted at pigmented tissue, so they don't work on white, grey or platinum blonde hair.

The bikini line–This area can be shaved or depilatory creams may be applied. This is a very sensitive area with folds of skins so be very careful to avoid nicks with razors and skin reactions with creams. Use with care, as if product gets into the vaginal area it can change the vaginal pH and lead to thrush and bacterial vaginosis.

Oral hygiene

Being busy with school, establishing a social life and increasing one's consumption of junk food can all have a detrimental effect on the teeth. Good oral hygiene practices should be part of every life from the moment a child grows his or her first tooth. Teeth brushing should be a twice daily activity.

Menstrual blood

Every woman's menstrual cycle is different. Some bleed for only a couple days and some for up to eight days. In addition, the heaviness of the bleeding varies from woman to woman and at different points in the period.

There are many different products available to absorb the blood during a period. Some women prefer one type over another and some use different products depending on the day of their period.

The two most common methods are pads that are put into the knickers and tampons that are put into the vagina. A third option is a type of cup that sits in the vagina to catch the blood and can be washed and reused. This is becoming more popular as women are becoming more aware of environmental issues and try to reduce the amount of waste produced. In addition, some women have concerns regarding Toxic Shock Syndrome, which has been linked to tampon use.

Menstrual pads

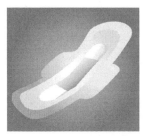

Menstrual pads are available in a wide variety of sizes, shapes, and brands. There are maxi pads for heavy days, and mini pads for light days. Some pads are thick and some are thin. Some even conform to the style of pants you wear. And some have 'wings' that fit over your pants to hold them in place. There are washable menstrual pads available also.

Tampons

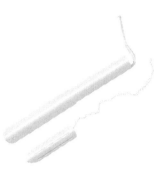

Today women have a wide choice of tampon brands. Some have cardboard applicators, some plastic, and others no applicator. There is much controversy about the safety of tampons and their possible connection to Toxic Shock Syndrome. Women who enjoy the convenience of tampons but who are concerned about possible health risks can find all-natural, organic, cotton tampons on several websites, as well as at local organic shops.

Disposable sanitary products should be wrapped and put in the bin or the sanitary bin provided in public toilets and not put down the toilet.

Toxic shock syndrome

Toxic shock syndrome (TSS) is a very rare, life–threatening infection that is most often associated with the use of tampons. TSS is caused by bacteria naturally present in the body in areas such as the nose, skin, or vagina. These bacteria produce toxins that generally cause only mild infections, if any. This is because most people have developed immunity to these toxins at some point in their lives. However, in rare instances people who are not immune to the toxins can have a severe reaction to them. TSS may rarely occur when the immune system is unable to combat the amount of toxins released during tampon use.

Symptoms of TSS develop suddenly and may include:
- high fever
- vomiting and/or diarrhoea
- a rash resembling a sunburn
- muscle aches
- redness of the eyes, mouth and/or throat
- seizures
- headaches
- low blood pressure.

If you feel you have these symptoms, you must seek medical advice immediately.

Menstrual cup

A menstrual cup is around two inches long and made from soft silicone rubber. It is worn internally like a tampon but collects menstrual fluid rather than absorbing. The cup is not a disposable product, so you only need to buy one.

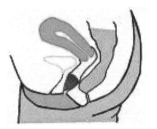 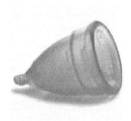

This cup will hold 30 mL of fluid, which is roughly one third of the average total produced each period. A light seal is formed with your vaginal walls, allowing menstrual fluid to pass into the cup without leakage or odour. You will probably need to empty your cup less frequently than you would need to replace pads or tampons.

 Check out the following websites for info on puberty and hygiene:
www.hygieneexpert.co.uk/CombatingPoorHygieneTeens.html
www.bbc.co.uk/science/humanbody/body/interactives/
lifecycle/teenagers

EMOTIONAL AND PSYCHOLOGICAL CHANGES IN PUBERTY

The 'tasks of adolescence'

We have considered the physical changes that occur in adolescence; in addition there are also psychological and social issues that young people typically grapple with during the teen years. Some sociologists have tried to identify the common issues that present during adolescence.

Recognised common issues are: forming identity, developing personal values, gaining independence socially and financially, body image, developing relationships with both sexes, developing thinking, acting in a socially acceptable manner and being responsible for own behaviour.

Forming a clear identity

The need to find an identity is a common driving force for teenagers. Young people often identify with certain reference groups. These may be typified by outward appearance such as clothing or hairstyles, or activities youth engage in like church groups, music performances, etc. Peer relationships are formed within these groups.

Individual rates of physical development can influence whether a young person is included in groups. A young person who is developing at a slower rate than his or her peers may still appear childlike and find it difficult to be included in the more 'advanced' groups.

Non-acceptance by the peer group can result in bullying, which causes psychological distress for the young person. Professionals working with young people should be aware that this may be an underlying problem in a young person's life. (*See below* for more information on bullying).

It can also be difficult to explore your identity if you are unable to become independent from parents and carers due to a disability.

Independence from parents is explored when forming an individual identity. Often 'parental' or 'adult' guidance is rejected, as young people want to explore issues themselves, with the common disbelief that anyone could have gone through what they are experiencing! There are many choices a young person has to make: which group to join, which belief system to choose, which career path to travel. Mixed with emerging sexuality, this can be overwhelming. Often young people move from one idea to another as they explore the possibilities. This can be confusing for the adults who observe these inconsistencies. However, it is important to support young people as they explore their identity. Such consistency from adults in their lives provides them with trustworthy role models.

Developing a personal value system

During adolescence the young person starts to develop thoughts and actions about what is right and wrong, rather than simply accepting parental beliefs. As they expand their social circles, young people will be faced with changing and sometimes conflicting values and standards of behaviour. Typically they will look to their peer groups to gain insight into how to behave. This can be complicated by conflicting approaches of peer groups and the young person's inexperience in making moral decisions. This may result in what the adult world would call delinquent behaviour or rebellious behaviour, yet is often simply experimentation with new possibilities. Adults should present sound, consistent values to young people. The young people will observe this, and these values will be incorporated into their decision-making processes. Value systems adopted can be simplistic, but they are equally valid in our complex society.

Gaining independence from parents

Parents will usually promote independence as a young person grows older. This depends on the parent-child relationship before adolescence. If the relationship has been overprotective, the young person will find it difficult to explore his or her own identity. Equally, young people may find it difficult to cope with the demands of being independent and will reject the opportunity, keeping 'childlike' behaviours.

A young person may move between adult and childlike behaviour, and this can be confusing for parents/carers and professionals. For example, an expanding social life can be dependant on parental transport and funding, or a developing sexual relationship may not go hand in hand with a responsible approach to contraception and safe sex.

Achieving financial and social independence

The social environment provides a filter through which the adolescent perceives the world. As they grow older, young people select and interpret these perceptions. A nurturing familial and social environment will provide support. As a young person gets older, parents may engender a practical approach to saving and budgeting by providing an allowance. Young people can take on part-time work and begin to have financial independence. This can be the cause of great conflict between parents/carers and teens. Teens have been used to parents providing clothes and recreational activities, yet as they grow older their tastes become more expensive and they perceive needs where parents may not. Conflict may also arise when young people prioritise casual work over study, preferring to be 'cash rich' currently rather than investing for future security.

Some groups, such as young people with illness or disability, may experience problems in achieving social and financial independence from parents. They may be restricted in their ability to travel independently or in jobs that are available to them.

Accepting a new body image

Adolescents have little control over their changing bodies. With puberty come spots, sweating, and body hair. To successfully accept a new body image, young people need to be able to adapt to these changes. Some adolescents can develop preoccupations with body image, which may result in problems such as anorexia nervosa and bulimia. It is not clear why some young people develop these problems and others do not; however, it could be due to culturally defined messages that are portrayed by the media about the 'ideal' body shape and weight. Young people may feel undue pressure to conform to these unnatural 'norms'. Some young people may not be ready for imminent adulthood and develop eating behaviours to try to stay thin and childlike (*see* Chapter 2 for further exploration of eating disorders).

Adolescents who have been sexually abused may be particularly confused about their emerging sexuality and sexual identity. An adult appearance may be associated with negative feelings. The young person may need support to re-evaluate these feelings and to learn to develop healthy and fulfilling sexual relationships.

Meanwhile, a hormonal rollercoaster can cause mood swings, volatile behaviour and a general lack of control over emotions. This can be an unpredictable and difficult time for teenagers.

Developing relationships with members of both sexes

Peer relationships become increasingly important during adolescence. Their role is often to provide a support mechanism and a reference group with which the young person can begin to identify. At first it is typical for a young person to form same-sex friendships; later on, same-sex relationships are formed commonly in a group; then even later teens will commonly pair off. Teens may struggle with issues such as sexuality, whether they are attractive to the opposite/same sex, and how to act in relationships.

Developing sexuality

It's a natural part of life to have sexual feelings. As people pass from childhood through adolescence to adulthood, sexual feelings develop and change. As previously discussed, during the teen years sexual feelings are awakened in new ways because of the hormonal and physical changes of puberty. Part of this development includes a person's sexual feelings and attractions. The term 'sexual orientation' refers to the gender to which a person is attracted. There are several types of sexual orientation that are commonly described:

- **heterosexual.** People who are heterosexual are romantically and physically attracted to members of the opposite sex: Heterosexual males are attracted to females, and heterosexual females are attracted to males. Heterosexuals are sometimes called 'straight'
- **homosexual.** People who are homosexual are romantically and physically attracted to people of the same sex: Females who are attracted to other females are lesbian; males who are attracted to other males are often known as gay (The term gay is sometimes also used to describe homosexual individuals of either gender.)
- **bisexual.** People who are bisexual are romantically and physically attracted to members of both sexes.

Thinking sexually about both the same sex and the opposite sex is quite common as people sort through their emerging sexual feelings. This type of imagining about people of the same or opposite sex doesn't necessarily mean that a person fits into a particular type of sexual orientation. Some teens may also experiment with sexual experiences, including those with members of the same sex, during the years they are exploring their own sexuality. These experiences, by themselves, do not necessarily mean that a person is gay or straight.

Do people choose their sexual orientation?

Most medical professionals believe that sexual orientation involves a complex mixture of biology, psychology, and environmental factors. A person's genes and inborn hormonal factors may play a role as well. These medical professionals believe that, in most cases, sexual orientation is not simply chosen. In some cases sexual orientation may be affected by the life experiences that a person has had.

There are lots of opinions and stereotypes about sexual orientation, and some of these can be hurtful to people of all orientations. For example, having a more 'feminine' appearance or interest does not mean that a man is gay. And having a more 'masculine' appearance doesn't mean a woman is lesbian. As with most things, making assumptions just based on looks can lead to the wrong conclusion.

What's it like for gay teens?

For many people who are gay or lesbian, it can feel like everyone is expected to be straight. Because of this, some gay and lesbian teens may feel different from their friends when the heterosexual people around them start talking about romantic feelings, dating and sex. They may feel like they have to pretend to feel things that they don't in order to fit in. They might feel they need to deny who they are or that they have to hide an important part of themselves.

These feelings, plus fears of prejudice, can lead people to keep their sexual orientation secret, even from friends and family. Some gay or lesbian teens tell a few accepting, supportive friends and family members about their sexual orientation. This is often called 'coming out'. Many lesbian, gay, and bisexual teens who come out to their friends and families are fully accepted by them and their communities. They feel comfortable about being attracted to someone of the same gender and don't feel anxious about it.

But not everyone has the same feelings or good support systems. People who feel they need to hide who they are or who fear rejection, discrimination, or violence can be at greater risk for emotional problems like anxiety and depression. Some gay teens without support systems can be at higher risk than heterosexual teens for dropping out of school, living on the streets, using alcohol and drugs, and even in some cases for attempting to harm themselves. These difficulties are thought to happen more frequently not directly because they are gay, but because gay and lesbian people are more likely to be misunderstood, socially isolated, or mistreated because of their sexual orientation.

Developing cognitive skills and abstract thought

At the same time that all these physical changes are occurring to a young person, the complexity of thought processes is developing. An ability to give consideration to a range of consequences and to reason develops, leading to logical and systematic decision-making. However, this is a process, and the teenage years are characterised by egocentric thought: the notion that what they are thinking and experiencing is completely new and unique to them! It is important to bear in mind when working with a group of teenagers that they will all be at different stages in this process.

Developing behaviour control and taking responsibility

Usually the peer group provides the main reference for behavioural choices for a young person. Sometimes the peer group influence may override a young person's parents, and the young person may be seen as exhibiting rebellious behaviour. Self-esteem and self-confidence influence a young person's ability to make independent behavioural choices. However, the strong desire to belong can influence a young person's choice of behaviour within a peer group. It is very important for the young person to feel accepted, and hence to conform to the group norm. This can range from the adolescent's choice of clothing to more risky behaviours such as drug taking.

Bullying

What is bullying? Bullying includes a wide variety of behaviors, but all involve a person or a group repeatedly trying to harm someone who is perceived to be weaker or more vulnerable. It can involve direct attacks such as hitting, threatening or intimidating, maliciously teasing and taunting, name-calling, making sexual remarks, and stealing or damaging belongings—or more subtle, indirect attacks such as spreading rumors or encouraging others to reject or exclude someone.

Bullying can lead teenagers to feel tense, anxious and afraid. If bullying continues for some time, it can begin to affect self-esteem and self-worth. It can increase social isolation, leading victims to become withdrawn and depressed, anxious and insecure. On rare occasions, it can lead to self-harm and even suicide.

Years later, long after the bullying has stopped, adults who were bullied as teens have higher levels of depression and poorer self-esteem than other adults.

Exploring bullying

Put the following numbered statements onto a card. Give one to each group member, or if in a larger group, give one card to each small group. Get each individual or small group to think about the statement, then share their thoughts and receive feedback. Note important points on flip-chart paper that can be displayed for the young people to see on in their own time.

Alternatively, stick three signs at three points in the room stating 'agree', 'disagree' or 'don't know'. Read out the statement and ask the group members to stand according to what they feel about the statement. Encourage discussion according to the group/individual response.

Statements about bullying

1 Bullying doesn't happen in our school/youth group.
2 Physical bullying is worse than name-calling.
3 Being left out is a form of bullying.
4 A lot of people are bullied but don't tell anyone.
5 Bullying is a one-off event.
6 Bullying is deliberately hurtful.
7 It's the fault of the victim: they should stand up for themselves.
8 Anyone can be bullied—or be a bully.
9 Bullying often happens on the playground.
10 Bullying happens more among girls than among boys.
11 I've seen people being bullied at school.
12 Bullying is a normal part of growing up; it doesn't hurt anyone.
13 Sticks and stones may break my bones, but words will never hurt me.
14 Everyone can help to stop bullying.

Bullying scenario

Ask the young people to volunteer to read the different parts in the following script, with accompanying actions if they wish. The pupils then read the situation again. After the pupils have read their lines, they 'freeze', and pupils in the 'audience' have the opportunity to ask the readers how they are feeling and why they are behaving in this way. If they wish, pupils from the audience can also volunteer to come up to the front, step into the shoes of the actors, and act out a different way of behaving (which would have a positive out-come for Mark—read on).

Sean: *(Trips up Mark as he comes into the classroom, grabs his bag and empties the contents onto the floor)* Oops—now that was care-less, wasn't it? Better pick it up quick before you get into a row. Mummy wouldn't like that, would she? Idiot!

Ian: *(Comes in just as Mark is picking up his things, and 'accidentally' bumps into him)* Oh sorry, Mark I didn't see you there! You'd better move—making the place look untidy! *(laughs)*

Maria: Yeah, come on, Mark, sit down and get your things out quick or you might lose your place as teacher's pet!

At this point the teacher walks in. Mark sits down quickly, next to Katy.

Katy: There's a funny smell around here, Maria, don't you think? Smells of swots ... I'd better move. *(leaves Mark sitting on his own)*

Ruth: *(Sitting behind Katy)* Honestly, they can't half be horrible! Why can't they leave him alone? Anyway, it'll probably be someone else next week! Hope it's not me!

Rob: *(Who also saw what happened)* I wish they'd give up—poor Mark! But then it's none of my business—best keep my nose out. Mark should stick up for himself.

Mark: *(Pretends to be studying his textbook)* I've had enough! What have I done to deserve this? They're all the same—nobody's willing to stand up for me! I hate this school!

For discussion

Emphasise that bullying is everyone's responsibility and that everyone has the right to feel safe and to be respected.
What can we do to ensure that this happens in practice?
   Some things we can do in a bullying situation are:
   • refuse to join in
   • tell the bullies to stop
   • be friendly towards the victim
   • tell a teacher or another responsible adult what's happening.

These activities were adapted from suggested workshops by the NSPCC.
   These and more can be found at: www.nspcc.org.uk/getinvolved/raise money/fundraisinginschools/defeatbullying/teaching_resources_wda50411. html

Tackling homophobic bullying

Dealing with discriminatory language and interactions

Discriminatory language can range from derogatory language to well-meaning but misplaced comments, as well as direct accusation. Derogatory language could be something such as 'that coat is so gay'. While the term can be understood to be derisive in this context, many pupils and staff members do not regard such usage as homophobic, as it is not directed at a person perceived to be homosexual. The young person may not have considered the meaning of this word and is simply using it as a derogatory term, however its use perpetuates the standpoint that gay is negative. A well-meaning professional may say, 'when did you decide to be gay?' demonstrating ignorance about sexual orientation, is another example.

   Society in general could be considered as heterosexist in that generally there is the expectation that someone is heterosexual unless they specifically state otherwise. Direct accusation is where a person or group is accused of being gay due to a range of 'reasons' usually when not conforming to group stereotype.

   So how do we tackle this language or action? The key is to be prepared in advance. These incidents tend to be spontaneous, so to have formulated a response in advance will put you in good stead. Although dealing with spontaneous instances is nerve-racking as you cannot predict how people will react to your challenge, the more it is done, the more confidence you will gain.

The first step is to interrupt the action/verbal insult. This should be done as soon as you become aware of it. In the first instance, gently challenge the language or the action that is a manifestation of bullying and not the belief from which you feel the insult or action may have come. This shows that bullying and discrimination will not be tolerated, yet does not humiliate the perpetrator and challenge core beliefs that would not be appropriate in a group setting.

Later on, find an opportunity to talk with the targeted person and the perpetrator individually. Offer the targeted person an opportunity to talk about the incident. Be prepared with information and resources that may be useful to the person such as reading materials, details of community organisations and support groups. Offer the same opportunity to the perpetrator. This is the place to explore from what motivation the action has come, e.g. hate, fear or seeking peer approval.

Finally, reflect on the incident yourself and how you dealt with it. Explore your own feelings. Talk it over with someone who can provide the support you need, particularly where feelings are not resolved, or simply to gain insight from another perspective. Explore how you may have dealt with it differently; this will be useful for future interactions. Above all, affirm yourself for intervening; remember why it is important to do so, and recognise that you have acted according to these healthy values.

National organisations

Stonewall—Stonewall works for equality and justice for lesbians, gay men and bisexuals. www.stonewall.org.uk

Broken Rainbow—Broken Rainbow is a UK-wide service offering support to lesbian, gay, bisexual and transgender victims and survivors of domestic violence and abuse. www.broken-rainbow.org.uk

The Lesbian and Gay Foundation—The LGF Helpline is available at 0845 3 30 30 30 (local call rate) from 6 p.m.–10 p.m. (staffed) and 10 p.m.–6 p.m. (automated system). www.lgf.org.uk

---

PROMOTING A POSITIVE ETHOS IN A GROUP OR INSTITUTION

Policy

It is important to look at the overall ethos of a group or institution to ensure that it tackles homophobic bullying. This should be both explicit, i.e. having an anti-homophobic bullying policy and implicit by looking at the language used in general policy material, i.e. ensuring resources used for group work contain inclusive images that challenge stereotypical ideas of gender and sexuality.

An anti-homophobic bullying 'policy' need not be long and wordy. For example:

- at ... we believe that homophobic bullying is unacceptable
- we adopt a zero-tolerance approach to homophobia and homophobic language
- we are developing opportunities to examine these issues. (Note: For schools this could be in Personal Social and Health Education (PSHE), and citizenship and youth groups could deliver workshops or invite external speakers.)

Training

Staff training is also a vital part of intervening against homophobic bullying. The same workshop can be used for both adults and young people to explore discriminatory attitudes and actions. In addition, staff should be aware how general reactions can perpetuate narrow definitions of what is 'typically' male and female. All professionals can play a vital role in challenging these stereotypical images simply by responding positively to children with the courage to be different. Staff should consider how they react to, for example, boys who prefer to dress up or girls who want to play with their male classmates. They should also reflect on how they deal with any negative reactions from other pupils to these choices.

Workshop

The aims of a workshop on discrimination should be to give the participants the opportunity to explore attitudes and their consequences in a safe space. It is more effective to discuss sexuality and homophobia within the broader context of equality, diversity, prejudice, stereotyping and discrimination. A session focusing solely on homophobia risks exposing young people who may already be targets of bullying.

Always establish ground rules at the onset. Facilitate this from the group so there is a sense of ownership rather than an imposed set of rules. This should make overt that this is a safe, confidential space for exploration of issues where group members respect each other and offer each other space to express and explore their feelings and belief systems. Having these ground rules written up on flip-chart paper is a useful tool to refer to during the workshop as needed.

A workshop could contain the following elements:

Exploring homophobia/bullying workshop

Ground rules:
- this group will respect people's individual experience
- this group will respect individual political choices
- members of the group will be open to each other's thoughts and feelings
- no question will be seen as 'wrong'
- discussions within the group will remain confidential
- phones will be put on silent
- one person may talk at a time
- respect time keeping.

Introduction
(Facilitator-led with flip chart note key words, events, phrases)
- What is discrimination?
- Give some examples of discrimination, either local or historical.
- Explore why these attitudes and actions are wrong/negative/ destructive.

Use of language
- Think of all the terms used that refer to someone's sexual orientation.

Brainstorm and discuss:
- are these positive or negative terms?
- how would a person feel if called these names? Can you draw parallels with bullying regarding race or gender, e.g. 'You run like a girl.'

Physical bullying and violence
- Why is difference sometimes threatening? How can it lead to bullying?

Split into smaller groups and consider the following events. Think about how this makes the group members feel. Do they consider this reasonable action? Why/why not?

Just after 6.30 p.m. on Friday 30 April 1999, the Admiral Duncan, a gay pub in London, was bombed by a young man who had also planted a nail bomb a few days earlier in Brixton and Brick Lane where the targets were members of London's Black and Bangladeshi communities.

In March 1997, 15-year-old Darren Steele killed himself after suffering five years of bullying. He was burnt with cigarettes, battered with schoolbooks and called 'poof' and 'gayboy' because he enjoyed cookery and drama lessons.

Conclusion
- What are some of the benefits of promoting acceptance, tolerance and challenging prejudice?
- How can we do this? (Think about language, policy, etc.)

Additional Information

www.teenagehealthfreak.org
Teen Health Website

CHAPTER 2

How do I look?

Body image during adolescence

INTRODUCTION

Body image is the mental picture we have about the way we think we look. It's how we feel about the size, shape, weight and look of our bodies.

For young people who are undergoing rapidly changing body shape, size and functioning, perception of body image is changing. This presents many challenges as adolescents work out where they fit in with society's perceived norms as well as their own goals and aspirations.

In addition, young people are bombarded with images in the media of what is perceived to be the 'ideal image'. The majority of us are naturally not like these images, and those with the ability to understand that this is not reality and that to have these body shapes does not necessarily equal a happy fulfilling life tend to develop a healthy body image. However, those who see these images as the ideal body image may struggle with their own body image and develop complex relationships with food and exercise; their self-esteem may suffer as well. Sometimes these problems can develop into complex mental health issues.

Going through puberty can amplify body image concerns. In addition, going through puberty later or earlier than peers can have an impact on body image as well as psychological health. Generally, early development for girls and late development for boys presents the greatest challenges to healthy body image.

This chapter will look at influences on body image and discuss eating disorders, steroid use, disabilities and chronic health conditions in relation to body image.

The influences

Right from childhood, where action figures and dolls have similar body shapes—tall and slender for female figures, and tall, slender and muscular for male figures—the body shapes advertised even by toys are not realistic. If Barbie were real, for example, her neck would be too long and thin to support the weight of her head, and her upper body proportions would make it difficult for her to walk upright. If Ken, her male counterpart, were real, his huge barrel chest and enormously thick neck would nearly preclude him from wearing a shirt.

The media are full of information about the nation's relationship with body weight. Prime-time television features programmes on how to make the best of your body shape, but more sinister are the makeover programmes that use radical surgery to 'improve' a person's looks. More specifically, there are interesting statistics on young people and their attitudes to their bodies.

The BBC reported a survey last year that found that half of young women would have surgery to improve their looks and a third of those who are a size 12 think they are overweight. BBC Radio 1's Newsbeat and 1xtra's TXU asked 25 000 people, mostly aged 17 to 34, how they felt about their bodies. Almost half the women surveyed said they had skipped a meal to lose weight, while about one in 10 had made themselves sick. The survey found two thirds of those who are size 14 also thought they were overweight or fat. Despite the celebrity emphasis on being size zero (UK size four), fewer than one in a hundred of those surveyed said they were that size.

Activity

- Find images of a size zero woman and a size 16+ woman; present these images to the group for discussion.
- What does the group think about the different images?
- Which size would they rather be? (If female)
- What do the boys think? Explore.

Young men also feel the pressure to look good. About one in five of those in their early 20s have taken protein supplements in a bid to help themselves bulk up, compared with one in 10 of those over age 35. And when asked to rate photos of differently shaped male bodies, almost 80% of men and 65% of women favoured a very muscular physique.

Activity

Find several images of very muscular men, from those with a regular workout routine to competitive body builders. Print off these images and discuss group and individual reactions and feelings.

For years, and more so recently, the entertainment and marketing industries have been blamed for causing eating disorders in adolescent and pre-teen girls. Opinion is that the constant bombardment of images and commercials portraying the "perfect" skinny body makes young girls feel inadequate, causing many to strive for the same physical perfection. The fashion industry has received much of the focus and blame in the past few months as some models have fallen ill as the result of eating disorders.

Activity

Compare and contrast
Find an image of a typical size zero catwalk model alongside the classic pin-up Marilyn Monroe, reputedly a size 14. Ask your group which is a more attractive, healthy image?

However, recent research points the finger in a completely different direction. It suggests that eating disorders such as anorexia and bulimia may be 'as inheritable as other psychiatric illnesses such as schizophrenia, depression, anxiety and obsessive-compulsive disorder.' Two chromosomes in particular (one and 10) have been linked to both anorexia and bulimia, and several other genes have been identified that may pre-dispose people to these eating disorders.

For some, this kind of information isn't entirely new. It has been a well-known fact in the medical community for decades that eating disorders are more common among families. Studies have revealed that if someone's mother or sister has suffered from anorexia, that person is 12 times more likely to develop the disorder herself.

Naturally there is no one cause for distorted body image; whilst the media plays a significant part in expectations for body image, there are those that may be genetically predisposed to developing eating disorders.

Activity

Exploring the influences on body image

Get your group to brainstorm what it thinks might be the influences on a young person's body image.

Suggestions could include:

- parents
- media
- genes
- friends
- peers
- goals and aspirations.

What situations might make the formation of a healthy body image more difficult?

Suggestions could include:

- disability
- chronic health conditions
- race
- stature
- fitness
- body mass.

Activity

Exploring body image

Form same-sex groups with four to five young people in each group. Give each group two sheets of paper and a marker.

- On one piece of paper, make a list of the parts of the body that people of your gender often feel dissatisfied with. Label your list **'Men often do not like ...'** or **'Women often do not like ...'**
- Using two or three magazines, find pictures of members of your sex that you think are attractive. Make a collage of these pictures or your own drawings on another piece of paper. Add words or phrases that describe an attractive member of your own sex.
- When you have finished the collage, tape both the list and the collage side by side on one of the walls.

Ask teens to walk around the room, read the lists, and look at the collages. Ask everyone to take a seat. Summarise what you see on the lists and ask thoughtful questions about what the lists and collages present. Consider the following discussion points:

Discussion:

Do you think that women or men are generally more satisfied with their bodies? Why?

Where do we get our ideas about what is attractive and what is not?

Did you find pictures that coincided with your ideas about what is attractive? If not, what were you looking for that you couldn't find?

Are you affected by other people's opinions about your body? How do you know what their opinions are?

Do media images influence how attractive or appealing we feel? Does the behaviour of people toward whom we are attracted influence how we feel?

Can we change some parts of our bodies? Which ones and how? Have we really changed when we change these parts of our bodies? Are we better people?

What parts of us can we not change? Does our inability to change some parts of our bodies mean we are unattractive?

What is it about us that is attractive and that does not rest on our appearance? *[If the young people do not suggest these things, be sure to bring them up: humour, intelligence, friendliness, kindness, tact, consideration, patience, determination, compassion, our ability to love and be loved, to be a good parent, student, employee, or employer, friend, neighbour]*

What things can teens do to feel better about their bodies? *[Answers should include supporting each other, paying less attention to media images, talking to a counsellor.]*

EATING DISORDERS

Women's preoccupation with the current beauty myth is evident in most cultures that have television and other media influences. Sadly, more and more women aspire to the stereotypical ideal. They are preoccupied with either getting thin or staying thin. For many young girls, this starts as early as primary school. These attitudes can develop into eating disorders.

Some might say that this is a form of violence that women do to themselves. Excessive dieting can not only lead to starvation by robbing the body of essential nutrients and thereby damaging the organs, in extreme cases it can cause death. The mindset also fosters a very unhealthy set of attitudes; these affect relationships, both now and in the future.

The two most common eating disorders are anorexia nervosa and bulimia. Anorexics pursue thinness through extreme dieting and excessive exercise, while bulimics eat out of control and then purge themselves by vomiting, fasting, taking laxatives and exercising.

Anorexia

Anorexia affects mostly girls, though there has been a rise in the number of boys who are reported as anorexic. The disorder generally begins in mid-teenage years, though children as young as nine are reported to be dieting and may be putting themselves at risk. A third of anorexics were overweight as children.

Anorexia is an eating disorder characterised by an obsessive desire to lose weight and a distorted body image. Though sufferers are painfully thin, they see themselves as fat and starve themselves to prevent weight gain. They may also use other methods to lose weight, like making themselves sick after eating, dosing themselves with laxatives or excessive exercise.

Activity

Look at these real-life quotes from people with eating disorders and discuss.

Source: www.livereal.com/psychology_arena/whats_the_problem/anorexia_quotes.htm

'It wasn't simply that I chose not to eat; I was forbidden to. Even thinking about forbidden foods brought punishment.... How dare you, this voice inside me would say. You greedy pig.'

'Nothing tastes as good as thin feels'

'Nothing matters when I'm thin'

'You will be tempted quite frequently, and you will have to choose whether you will enjoy your self hugely in the 20 minutes or so that you will be consuming the excess calories, or whether you will dislike yourself for two or three days, for your lack of willpower'

'I have a rule when I weigh myself; if I've gained, I starve for the rest of the day. But if I've lost, I starve too.'

'An imperfect body reflects an imperfect person ...'

Weight loss

Anorexics appear painfully thin. Girls will often wear loose-fitting and lay-ered clothes to hide their thinness. Layers of woolly clothing may also help to keep them warm as the drastic change in weight often causes a drop in body temperature.

As their stomach contracts due to the low food intake, sufferers complain of abdominal pains after eating. Lack of food can cause bouts of constipation and large quantities of laxatives may be taken, partly for constipation and to get rid of any food they have eaten.

When body weight falls below a certain level, anorexics find that their periods stop. If anorexia occurs before puberty, it will stop its onset. Skin becomes dry, nails become brittle and a growth of downy hair may appear on the face.

Changes in eating habits

A teenager suffering from anorexia may skip family meals, claiming that he or she has already eaten. Anorexics avoid eating with others and snatch 'meals' at odd moments of the day. Food may be cut up into small portions and pushed around the plate. Bulky but low-calorie food, such as celery or lettuce, is piled high and substituted for more substantial food.

Changes in behaviour

Anorexics may exercise excessively, though their weight loss makes them weak and easily tired. They may count calories obsessively, read slimming magazines avidly and weigh themselves several times a day. Surprisingly, though they eat very little, anorexics are preoccupied with food and often love to cook for other people.

Seek professional help

Anorexia is a serious illness and, in a small percentage of cases, fatal. Argument and persuasion from family members will not help. The underlying condition is a form of mental illness and the sufferer needs professional help—the earlier, the better. Provide support and encouragement without intruding. For many anorexics, it appears that their weight is the only area of their life in which they have control. They may therefore be very resistant to getting treatment, which they feel will take away their control. It is vital to approach the matter delicately.

Discuss the following case studies

Case study 1

Miranda developed anorexia nervosa when she was 16. Fifteen years later she has recovered but is a self-confessed habitually mindful person about what she eats.

'I was a shy and apparently very bright teenager, the kind of girl that tried to please everyone. I was pretty and not fat—just had that normal puppy fat you have.

'I remember my father (who was joking) telling me maybe I was a little chubby. I took him seriously. I started dieting and didn't stop. Eventually my periods stopped. I was obsessed. I weighed my food all the time and did things like put my daily ration into small containers. I exercised—even in the bathroom. I was five feet nine tall and weighed less than 45 kilos. I ended up in hospital and on a drip for two weeks. It took a long time and a lot of help for me to face my problem.'

Source: www.hcf.com.au/Services/eating-disorders.asp

Case study 2

For Cora Healy, 28, anorexia was triggered by the prospect of leaving behind the security of secondary school.

'The pressure was on in sixth year; everyone knew what they wanted to do and I didn't know at all', she recalls. Her anxiety about the future found an outlet in a dislike of her own body. She began to limit her food intake, while exercising vigorously. 'Normal food turned to healthy food and then fewer calories. After a while, I'd only eat apples.'

Before long, she had lost a stone from her petite size eight frame. The well-intentioned intervention of her parents—involving counsellors and hypnotists—only made the teenager angry. 'The more it was made into an issue', she says, 'the more I wanted to control it. It was my little crutch to get me through that stage in my life.'

Source: www.independent.ie/topics/Cora+Healy

Additional resources

beat—Eating Disorders Association
www.b-eat.co.uk

Boys Get Anorexia Too
www.boyanorexia.com

Bulimia

Like teenagers with anorexia, teens with bulimia have great concern with weight and shape. Teenagers with bulimia regularly (at least twice a week) engage in overeating-even when not hungry. This is followed by guilt and anxiety and an attempt to remove the food from the body to avoid weight gain. Undoing the consequences of eating too much may involve self-induced vomiting, laxative use, diuretics, or enemas. Adolescents with bulimia may periodically skip meals, restrict food or engage in over-exercising. In spite of this, most people with bulimia are of normal weight.

Many people with bulimia have other behavioural and mental health problems, such as impulsivity, depression, self-inflicting harm through cutting and burning, and substance abuse problems. Over time, bulimic behaviours can result in physical problems. Some of these are swollen salivary glands, electrolyte and mineral imbalances, long-lasting disruption of normal bowel function, erosion of the dental enamel, and rarely, tearing or rupturing of the oesophagus or stomach or heart irregularities.

Bulimia is not generally seen in younger children and in general, has an older age of onset than anorexia (late teens and 20s).

Examples of media personalities with eating disorders

Kelly Clarkson—The 'American Idol' winner struggled with bulimia for six months until friends discovered her secret and begged her to get help.

Posh Spice—Having denied having an eating disorder in the past, September of 2001 found Posh Spice openly admitting to struggling with anorexia. She shared her obsession with her physical appearance and her severe dieting habits.

Britney Spears—The troubled singer has a binge personality and is very compulsive. She does mega workouts and watches what she eats for a few months, then she'll return to her binging behaviour.

Geri Halliwell—Singer Geri Halliwell (formerly Ginger Spice from the Spice Girls) publicly admitted suffering from bulimia and binge eating for several years. 'I realised I couldn't control this monster anymore. I needed to find help. There are lots of people who want to help and you really CAN'T fight this one on your own.'

Source: http://caringonline.com/eatdis/people.htm

Additional resources

There are 3 excellent videos on the NHS Choices website about teenagers and eating disorders:

Anorexia real story
http://tinyurl.com/yzycmux

Eating disorders: friends
http://tinyurl.com/y929lzo

Eating disorders: teenagers
http://tinyurl.com/yce8gwy

Eating disorders and young men

Historically, eating disorders have been almost exclusively associated with females. However, there are a growing number of young men being identified with these disorders. Experts say that males with eating disorders tend to obsess over particular body types, rather than weight, and that these types can vary drastically. One may want to be lean, another extremely muscular.

Males tend to develop eating disorders in connection with athletic performance. They typically obsess about their percentage of body fat. They develop food phobias based on what will and won't give them a competitive edge. This fixation with performance often leads them to other drastic measures such as steroids and compulsive exercise. In addition, athletic teams and coaches often encourage unhealthy eating and exercise practices as a part of physical conditioning. Sports that require weigh-ins, such as wrestling and boxing, are the most susceptible to extreme eating and exercise regimens.

 Watch this video on male anorexia on the NHS Choices website: http://tinyurl.com/yjrogo5

Anabolic steroids

Anabolic steroids are associated with sports, bodybuilding and body shaping. Anabolic steroids are used because of their ability to improve performance by increasing muscle mass and decreasing body fat, so their use depends on the type of sport undertaken.

It is believed that anabolic steroid use is widespread in competitive body-building. Steroid use in sport is illegal and international athletes are tested to prevent some gaining an unfair advantage.

Anabolic steroids are also used, especially by men, to change their body shape towards a more muscular physique.

In medicine, steroids are used for various conditions such as delayed puberty, some types of impotence, wasting of the body due to such conditions as HIV, some types of anaemia and osteoporosis. Anabolic steroids can be taken orally, by injection or in creams or gels. Dosages prescribed by doctors will depend on the medical condition, its severity and the age of the patient.

In the illegal use of this group of steroids, dosages are highly variable and can be 10 to 40 to sometimes even 100 times higher than the recommended dosage.

Side effects and complications of anabolic steroid abuse

The side effects of anabolic steroids are serious and not uncommon. In general, oral anabolic steroids have more side effects—some are reversible, but some can cause permanent damage.

- Anabolic steroids reduce the liver's excretory function. The liver can suffer from a bleeding cystic condition that is potentially fatal. Use of steroids has also been linked to liver cancer.
- Anabolic steroids can cause cardiovascular system damage, problems with blood pressure and lipoproteins such as cholesterol. There is some evidence that anabolic steroids can cause structural changes to the heart and that heart disease and strokes are possible with anabolic steroids, especially oral types of the drug.
- Increased erectile dysfunction and impotence are common, even though sexual desire is increased.
- Gynecomastia (breast growth) may occur, which is a condition that is generally irreversible.
- Atrophy or shrinkage of the testicles can occur and is reported usually with high-dose usage of anabolic steroids.

Source: http://menshealth.about.com/cs/fitness/a/anab_steroids.htm

Young men and body image

Show photos of men from magazine ads.

Ask students:

- what messages are being given to men through these images? How are they different from the messages that we get from the images of women that we see?
- do you think that men are also pressured to look a certain way?

There is pressure for men or boys to look like these images, but mostly, they face pressure to do or act in certain ways, rather than look a certain way. Physical ability is very important in becoming a man, and it is often used to prove one's manhood. From films, sports activities, men get the message that to be a real man, you must be the toughest.

- Name some media role models who send this type of message.
- What does the group think men physically have to do to prove that they are 'real men'? Is this actually the case?

Body dysmorphic disorder

Body dysmorphic disorder (BDD) is a mental illness. People who have this illness constantly worry about the way they look. They may think something that isn't there, or that others don't even notice, is a serious defect. The severity of BDD varies. For example, some people know their feelings aren't rational or justified, while others are almost delusional in their conviction.

The preoccupation can be so extreme that the affected person has trouble functioning at work, school or in social situations. Any part of the body can be targeted. It is thought that about 1% of the population may have BDD, with men and women equally affected. BDD usually starts in the teenage years, when concern over physical appearance is common.

Common areas of concern include:
• facial skin
• face, including the size or shape of the eyes, nose, ears and lips
• size or shape of virtually any body part including buttocks, thighs, abdomen, legs, breasts and genitals
• overall size and shape of the body
• symmetry of the body or particular body parts.

Symptoms

Symptoms can vary according to which body part (or parts) are targeted, but general symptoms of BDD include:
• thinking about the perceived defect for hours every day
• worrying about their failure to match the 'physical perfection' of models and celebrities
• distress about their preoccupation
• constantly asking trusted loved ones for reassurance about their looks, but not believing the answer
• constantly looking at their reflection, or taking pains to avoid catching their reflection (for example, throwing away or covering up mirrors)
• constant dieting and over-exercising
• grooming to excess—for example, shaving the same patch of skin over and over
• avoiding any situation they feel will call attention to their defect. In extreme cases, this can mean never leaving home
• taking great pains to hide or camouflage the 'defect'
• squeezing or picking at skin blemishes for hours on end
• wanting dermatological treatment or cosmetic surgery, even when professionals believe the treatment is unnecessary

- repeat cosmetic surgery procedures, especially if the same body part is being 'improved' with each procedure
- depression and anxiety, including suicidal thoughts.

The cause of BDD is unknown. Theories include:
- a person with BDD has a genetic tendency to develop this type of mental illness. The trigger may be the stress of adolescence
- particular drugs, such as ecstasy, may trigger onset in susceptible people
- BDD could be caused by chemical imbalances in the brain
- a person with low self-esteem who has impossible standards of perfection judges some part of their body as ugly, and over time, this behaviour becomes more and more compulsive
- western society's narrow standards of beauty may trigger BDD in vulnerable people.

BODY IMAGE AND DISABILITY

Body image evolves gradually and reflects interactive forces exerted by sensory, interpersonal, environmental and temporal factors. Disability, with its impact on physical appearance, functional capabilities, experience of pain, and social roles can alter and even distort one's body image and self-concept. Successful adaptation to disability is said to reflect the integration of physical and sensory changes into a transformed body image and self-perception. Unsuccessful adaptation, in contrast, is evidenced by experiences of physical and psychiatric symptoms such as feelings of anxiety and depression, pain, chronic fatigue, social withdrawal and cognitive distortions.

One's self-concept and self-identity are linked to body image and are often seen as conscious, social derivatives of it. However, self-concept and self-identity may be discordant for many individuals with visible disabilities. The sense of self that is privately owned and outwardly presented may be denied in social interactions with others who respond to the person as 'disabled' first, losing sense of the person's real self. As a consequence, the person's self-esteem gradually shows signs of erosion and negative self-perceptions following such encounters. The challenges for adolescents with a disability can be similar to those with a chronic health condition.

Activity

Present images of people with disabilities to the group and discuss some of the assumptions that may be made when meeting a person with an obvious disability. Gently explore attitudes and assumptions.

BODY IMAGE AND CHRONIC HEALTH CONDITIONS

A young person with a chronic illness may be affected not just physically, but also emotionally, socially and sometimes even financially. The way a person is affected by a chronic illness depends on the particular illness and how it affects the body, how severe it is, and the kinds of treatments that might be involved.

Because the teen years are all about fitting in, it can be hard to feel different around friends and classmates. Many people with chronic illnesses are tempted to try to keep their condition secret. Sometimes, though, trying to hide a condition can cause its own troubles. For example, for a young teen with Crohn's disease, some of the necessary medications may make the young person look puffy. Classmates may start teasing the adolescent about gaining weight. However, when teens with chronic conditions explain their conditions to others, they may be surprised at how accepting classmates are.

There's no doubt the teen years can be a more challenging time to deal with a health condition. In addition to the social pressures to fit in, it's a time of learning about and understanding changing bodies. At a time when it's natural to be concerned with body image, it is hard to feel different.

The chronic disorder, treatments, hospitalizations and surgery (when necessary) all intensify concerns about physical appearance, interfere with the process of gaining independence, and disrupt evolving relationships with parents and friends. Also, adolescent developmental issues can complicate a teen's transition toward taking responsibility for managing their illness and learning to comply with recommended treatment.

Even teens who have lived with an illness since childhood can feel the pull of wanting to lead a 'normal' life in which they don't need medicine, have any limitations, or have to care for themselves in any special way. This is a perfectly natural reaction. Sometimes teens who have learned to manage their illness feel so healthy and strong that they wonder whether they need to keep following their disease management program. Unfortunately, this can have disastrous results if, for example, medication isn't taken.

CHALLENGES FOR ADOLESCENTS WITH A CHRONIC HEALTH CONDITION

Body image issues

Adolescents normally are focused on the physical changes occurring in their bodies. Chronic illness intensifies these concerns with fears or distortions related to their illness (such as the fear a surgical scar will interfere with physical attractiveness or the ability to wear certain clothes).

• Encourage adolescents to share their concerns related to their body and how it may be affected by their illness or treatment.

- Inform adolescents about anticipated physical effects of medications and treatment.
- Encourage discussion about ways to reduce or cope with the effects.

Developing independence

Chronic illness frequently interferes with an adolescent becoming less dependent on his or her parents. Parents of chronically ill adolescents often are more resistant to their child's efforts to act independently. Some ways to address this conflict, while still addressing the healthcare needs of the chronic illness, include the following:

- involve the young person in health-related discussions (such as concerns about the adolescent's illness or treatment choices)
- teach young people self-care skills related to their illness
- encourage young people to monitor and manage their own treatment needs as much as possible
- encourage the development of coping skills to address problems or concerns that might arise related to their illness.

Relationships with peers

Chronic illness and treatment often interfere with time spent with peers or at school, which is a teenager's primary social environment.
To address these concerns:

- encourage spending time with friends as much as possible
- discuss concerns about what to share with friends
- help find ways to respond if teased by peers
- encourage humour
- encourage/assist friends in being supportive.

DRUGS, ALCOHOL AND CHRONIC ILLNESS

Alcohol and recreational drug use can contribute to illness in teens with chronic illness and may interact adversely with prescribed medications.

RELATIONSHIPS AND CONTRACEPTION

Whereas some chronic conditions are associated with impaired fertility from the disease itself (e.g. male adolescents with cystic fibrosis) or from the treatment (e.g. survivors of certain childhood cancers), most chronic illnesses do not impair libido or fertility. Therefore, advice on effective contraception is extremely important. Although care must be taken in prescribing hormonal contraception to teenaged girls with a medical illness, most contraceptive methods are safer than pregnancy itself. Such teens should also be counselled about the necessity of carefully planning pregnancies to minimize harm to the foetus from medications and treatments.

 This website offers short film clips of young people discussing various aspects of their chronic health condition: www.healthtalkonline.org

Being aware of young people's perceived body image

Given that concerns over body image are common and sociocultural messages regarding body shape and size are continuous and unavoidable, it is wise to work with young people to foster a healthy body image. This can be done through listening and asking gentle questions.

Listen

Listen to young people talk about their health or any particular health concern; think about whether their concerns may be body image related or affecting their behaviours.

Young people may talk about wanting to lose weight or ask for weight loss advice; use this opportunity to discuss body image, healthy weight and shape, media influences, etc.

Young people may talk about a particular diet; again, use this opportunity to provide them with nutritionally sound information about myths, misinformation and dangers related to fad diets.

Young people may speak in a subtle or a strong way about a disliked part of the body or a concern about eating or food; use their comments as a starting point from which to explore their perception of their body and whether or not they are accurate.

Be attentive in general. A young person may make a brief comment that could serve as a terrific entrance into a valuable conversation about body image.

Ask questions
1 Bring questions about body image into your usual conversation.
2 Ask about body image concerns you think their friends have.
3 Ask on a regular basis, starting from before puberty and into adulthood.
4 With a more formal group, try a brief questionnaire from which to begin conversation.
5 Ask young people what the best questions are.

Some suggestions:

1 Are you concerned about your weight, shape or size at all? Do you think your friends are concerned about their weight?
2 Do you know that diets are the worst way to lose or maintain weight? Have you ever dieted? Why?
3 Do you know how to tell if you are too thin or too heavy or just right? How do you feel right now?
4 What would you do if you had a problem with your eating or if you were concerned a friend had a problem? Do you know anyone who has a problem with their eating? Have you talked to them about it?
5 Do you follow any special diet?
6 Do you ever take any pills to control your appetite or your weight? Does anyone you know do this?
7 What kind of exercise do you do? Why do you do it?

Have resources available for young people who do have body image issues or concerns. Have accurate, young people oriented resources available to read, look up on the net, or find in a library. Encourage young people to continue having conversations about these issues, either with you, their parents or another health professional. Encourage young people to be media literate to better handle the challenge of media stereotypes. Know which health professionals or clinics in your area treat eating disorders and understand their referral and screening process so you can make a referral if necessary.

Exploring gender stereotypes and body image

Write **Act Like a Man** at the top of the flip-chart paper and record student responses. (Note: begin by directing the question to the boys. The girls can then be encouraged to respond. Attempt to record students' own choice of words. If their responses are too wordy, ask them to simplify for display purposes (e.g. men don't cry, men are tough, men are strong). Draw a box around the entire list.

This is the ***Act Like a Man*** box. Inside the box is a list of attitudes and behaviours that boys are pressured to adopt in the process of becoming men in our society. Men and boys are not born this way; these roles are learned.

Next, write **Be Ladylike** at the top of another sheet of flip-chart paper and record student responses. As with the boys, begin by directing questions to the girls, then encourage boys to respond (e.g. girls are polite, girls are neat, girls are passive). Draw a box around this list.

This is the ***Be Ladylike*** box. It's full of stereotypes, just like the Act Like a Man box. Its walls of conformity are just as restrictive. Women also learn to conform to very specific role expectations as they grow up in our society.

Learning gender roles

Where do we learn these gender roles? (Discussion prompts: Who teach us these stereotypes—people in entertainment? Sports? Media? When the students respond 'TV' or 'films', ask for specific examples to list.)

- Write these responses down the left side, outside the box. You may draw arrows to illustrate how these influences reinforce the walls of the stereotype box.

How stereotypes are reinforced

- What names or put-downs are directed at boys when they don't fit the box? What names are women called if they step out of the stereotype box?
- Allow students to be blunt with their slang in this educational context.

- Write the names along the bottom of the appropriate box. You may draw arrows to illustrate how they reinforce the wall of the stereotype box.
- How do these labels and names reinforce the stereotype box?
- How does it feel when we are called these names?
- What do you think the person who is using these put-downs is feeling?

(These names are used in order to hurt people emotionally, and we react by retreating to the "safety" of the stereotype box.)

Evaluating the gender stereotypes
- How many boys in the class have never cried? Put your hands up. Does this mean that those of you who didn't put up your hands are wimps, nerds, etc.?
- What about the girls; how many want to be passive, etc.?

Stereotypes are destructive because they limit our potential. This is not to say that it's wrong for guys to like sports or fix cars or for girls to enjoy cooking (cite other examples from the list). (Note: It is important to make this point in order to be sensitive to boys or girls who may feel defensive.) The problem is that we are told that we must perform these roles in order to fit in. It is important for all of us to make our own decisions about what we do.

What are some situations where you may be pressured to 'act like a man' or 'be a lady'? (e.g. for boys, friends may tell you to try a cigarette or participate in a risky activity, to prove that you're 'tough', or for girls, you might be prevented from playing a certain sport or you might let someone bully you into doing something that you don't want to do, because it isn't 'ladylike' to argue or be assertive.)

- How might these stereotypes lead to violence? (e.g. boys might be expected to 'fight it out', rather than 'talk it out', and girls might be expected to put up with bullying rather than be assertive.)

CHAPTER 3

Mental health

Young people with mental health problems can find it difficult to function well in society, find it hard to form relationships and are also more likely to smoke, drink alcohol and use cannabis, with the linked negative consequences.

There is evidence that more mental health problems are being diagnosed in young people. Some believe, however, this is due in part to an increasing trend towards medicalising distress: classifying ordinary, often transient problems as illness. So whilst we do not want to label young people with mental health problems, we should be mindful of some of the stresses that may be impacting a young person and help them to identify coping strategies early on, before problems develop.

It is estimated that one in 10 children aged five to 15 has a mental health problem. Mental health problems are more common in boys than girls; however, by the age of 16 to 17 there is no difference between the sexes.

This chapter aims to explore some of the possible predisposing factors to mental health issues for young people, define some of the most common disorders affecting young people, look at what techniques professionals working with young people can use to help equip them to deal with life stresses and explore what agencies professionals can refer young people to when further support is needed.

The mental health act

Most people suffering from a mental health issue are supported informally through voluntary agencies, primary care and hospitals. In some cases, for the protection of self and society, individuals are restrained against their will for monitoring and treatment. The Mental Health Act 1983 governs the admission of people to psychiatric hospital against their will and details their rights while detained plus their discharge from hospital and aftercare. The Act applies in England and Wales.

The Mental Health Act 1983 is, like any other Act of Parliament, divided into Sections. This has coined the term 'being sectioned' to mean being compulsorily admitted to hospital.

There is no lower age limit to the Mental Health Act 1983 and there are no specific provisions in the Act relating to children. In theory, children and young people may be treated or compulsorily detained under it, but in practice very young children are not detained under the Act, with the majority being admitted as 'informal' patients by their parents.

Details of the Mental Health Act can be found on the Mind website at the following address: www.mind.org.uk/Information/Legal/OGMHA.htm

CHILD AND ADOLESCENT MENTAL HEALTH

Resilience and social and emotional skills are important for young people to avoid mental health problems.

Social and emotional skills comprise a wide range of attitudes, beliefs, and levels of understanding, including young people's self-awareness; their ability to manage their feelings; their motivations; their level of empathy with others; and their social skills. They help to shape young people's self-esteem, how they feel about themselves, how they feel about others from different backgrounds, and the extent to which they take control over their own lives.'

These skills directly affect how young people learn and achieve, their success in the labour market and the likelihood they will experience poorer outcomes such as becoming a teenage parent or being involved in crime.

WHAT CAN BE THE PREDISPOSING FACTORS TOWARDS MENTAL ILL HEALTH IN YOUNG PEOPLE?

Before considering different disorders, let's examine what these factors can be. The following list is extensive yet not exhaustive and gives a feel of the manifold issues that can lead to mental health issues.

• Important life events	• Failure
• Stress	• Problems of discipline
• Lack of order	• Intellectually disabled/language problems
• Learned behaviour	
• Personality/temperament	• Creative people are often misunderstood and labelled
• Problems of identity	
• Individuals 'fitting' society's values	• World environment, e.g. threat of war
• Lack of support: community/ school	• Geographical isolation
	• Traumatic events; loss; personal grief
• Lack of rewarding, energetic activities e.g. sport, leisure activities, youth	• Lack of experiential learning
	• Self-esteem
• Clubs	• Alienation: isolation
• Risk-taking	• Drugs and alcohol
• Parent alcoholism	• Sexuality
• Developmental/transitional issues	• Cultural differences
	• Incarceration
• Physiological problems; genetic causes	• Child-rearing practices
	• Poor role models
• The expectation to behave like adults before they are ready	• Single parent/step-parents
	• Divorce/separation
• 'Authority': rebellion	• Transient families
• Responsibility	• Fostering, adoption
• Poor education	• Parent psychopathology
• Unemployment	• Rejection
• Poverty	• Lack of support
• Homelessness	• Violence
• Current economic climate	• Physical and sexual abuse; neglect
• Communication	• Society: pressure to conform to the 'me' society, materialism
• Learning problems	
	• Peer issues/relationships

Source: **Mental Health and Young People:** A report into the nature of mental health problems experienced by young people and implications for service provision: A report to the National Youth Affairs Research Scheme (NYARS), prepared by Michael Sawyer, David Meldrum, Bruce Tonge, and Jennifer Clark, 1992. www.acys.utas.edu.au/nyars/mental/index.html

As you can see, predisposing factors are manifold and do not in themselves cause mental ill-health; this is where resilience influences a young person's ability to cope when faced with challenging life events.

Some issues are well-recognised as areas that can influence mental health; these are examined in more detail below.

Family break-up

People experience divorce, separation or relationship breakdown in different ways. Many children or young people feel loss, anger and guilt, whereas others may actually benefit, particularly if they have been removed from situations of long-standing conflict. The golden rule mentioned by children who have been through the breakdown of a parent's relationship is to talk about it. Young people dislike being kept in the dark, and need to be told the truth.

There is a significant link between the level of involvement by fathers and boys being in trouble with the police. Boys with little or no involvement from their father are more likely to offend; highly involved fathers are a major factor in boys' general wellbeing, protecting them against depression.

	Additional resources Know someone experiencing family breakup? Tell them about the excellent website It's Not Your Fault by Action for Children: www.itsnotyourfault.org
	For more information on surviving family break-up, read the children's section at: www.divorceaid.co.uk/child/children.htm

	Keeping a diary You could suggest that a young person experiencing family break-up keep a diary. This is helpful in several ways: it is an outlet for the young person's feelings, and over time they will hopefully see an improvement in the situation and how they are coping with it.

Fostering and adoption

A study of the prevalence of mental disorders in children aged five to 10 who were looked after by local authorities showed that they were five times more likely to have a mental health problem than children in private households.

Unresolved anxieties about identity may underlie mental health problems in some adopted children, especially if their adoptive parents are reluctant to talk about the situation. It is generally accepted that all adopted children should be told about their adoption as soon as they are able to understand. Many adopted people have a yearning to meet their birth parents and, since the Children's Act 1975 (which gave them access to their original birth certificates), many have been able to do so.

Additional resources

Young people struggling in foster care or who are adopted may gain some support from the following websites:
www.fosterclub.com
http://au.reachout.com/find/articles/adoption-coping-with-being-adopted

Bullying

Bullied children are six times more likely to contemplate suicide than those who are not bullied. Some children are badly bullied to the point that it affects their education, relationships and even their prospects for jobs in later life. Young people who identify themselves as lesbian, gay or bisexual have been found to be more susceptible to bullying at school.

There are several types of bullying, and it can take the following forms:

- verbal bullying—name calling, spreading rumours, sarcasm
- emotional bullying—exclusion from the group, ridicule, humiliation, tormenting
- physical violence
- threats
- racism—taunts, gestures
- sexual intimidation—unwanted comments or physical contact
- cyberbullying—bullying through social networking websites.

The NHS Choices website has good information about bullying:
www.nhs.uk/livewell/bullying/pages/bullyinghome.aspx

See Chapter 1 for more information on bullying.

There is a useful booklet about how to deal with bullying for young people from Kidscape. Available from the following website as a PDF:
www.kidscape.org.uk/assets/downloads/ksbeatbullying.pdf

Additional resources

See how other young people have dealt with bullying via Dr Ann's advice pages on the Teenage Health Freak website: www.doctorann.org/index/results.asp?keyword=Bullying

Bullying discussion

- Get individuals within the group to put down on Post-it notes what they think bullying is; come up with a definition.
- Ask if anyone can give examples of bullying; discuss.
- Ask why they think people get bullied and what they think makes someone a bully.
- Ask what the effects can be on someone who is bullied.
- Take and make suggestions of what a young person could do if being bullied, e.g. tell a trusted adult, ignore or avoid the bully, etc.

Cyberbullying

Cyberbullying is when someone uses technology, like the Internet or a mobile phone, to deliberately hurt, humiliate, harass or threaten someone else.

Different ways in which people cyberbully include:

Sending nasty text messages or horrible emails, posting hurtful comments on social networking sites, making prank calls, putting up bullying photos or videos onto the Internet and spreading these photos or videos, posting links to hate sites, and bullying in blogs, chat rooms, virtual worlds or on gaming sites.

Some of the effects of cyberbullying are: a lack of self confidence, low self-esteem, depression, not wanting to go on the Internet, becoming upset or angry, not wanting to go to school, and more serious effects, like self-harm.

Explore with the group:
- why cyberbullying might be worse than other types of bullying
- why it's not such a good idea to meet up with someone you meet online
- why victims of cyberbullying feel like there is no escape—even at home or on holiday, etc.
- the fact that anyone can be cyberbullied if they have access to a mobile or a computer.

Tips for safer surfing:

- tell someone you trust that you are being cyberbullied
- report any cyberbullying, whether it's targeted at you or not
- never respond/retaliate as this can make things worse. It may be difficult not to, but try to ignore it
- block the cyberbullies from contacting you
- save any offensive emails/texts as this can be used to trace them if necessary
- tell your parents/carers that you are being cyberbullied—if they don't know, they can't help you
- if you are continuously cyberbullied, consider changing your user ID
- don't post any personal details online
- don't let anyone know your password—even friends
- think carefully before you post any information
- never upload personal photos of yourself online for safety reasons
- register on the site http://cybermentors.org.uk to gain support from peers
- don't allow these tips to hinder your enjoyment—but allow them to enhance your online experience.

Source: http://cybermentors.org.uk

Additional resources

CyberMentors (http://cybermentors.org.uk) is a website where young people can go if they are being bullied, cyberbullied or maybe just going through a rough time. It is a resource that offers young people support and guidance from peers as well as trained professionals. All CyberMentors are aged 11 to 25 and have all been trained by an organisation called Beatbullying to be online (and offline) Peer Mentors. CyberMentors form relationships with the young people who register by chatting to them and offering assistance. The target audience of the website is young people aged eight to 16. Many schools are now signing up for this service to make sure their pupils are ready to get help if they need it. Everything is kept confidential, unless there is a safeguarding issue.

Source: www.beatbullying.org

Young carers

Tasks undertaken by young carers are many and varied and include housework, personal care for those they look after, companionship and emotional support.

The stress of caring may have a long-term impact on the mental health of the child or young person.

'Young Carers in the UK: the 2004 report' highlights some of the negative impacts of the caring role as:

- limited opportunities for social and leisure activities
- limited horizons and aspirations
- difficulty in relating to their peers because of different experiences and maturity levels. This can often lead to bullying
- isolation—a feeling of exclusion and being an outsider
- stigma by association—children can be victimised and bullied because a family member is different
- fear of what professionals might do—that someone may be removed from the home
- living with silence and secrets—hiding the family situation from others
- health problems, both physical and mental
- emotional difficulties—from adopting a role that is beyond their developmental ability or from seeing a loved one in pain, or in the case of mental ill health the person they are caring for may be irrational and unpredictable
- educational problems—missing school, being tired and distracted when at school, not completing homework. Many leave with low grades or no qualifications.

Source: Carers UK. *Young Carers in the UK: the 2004 report.* London EC1A 4JT; 20/25 Glasshouse Yard; 2004.

Identifying a young carer

- Often late or missing days or weeks of school for no apparent reason.
- Often tired or withdrawn.
- Difficulty joining in extra-curricular activities.
- Isolated or a victim of bullying—either because of the situation in the family or because they lack social skills when with their peers; in contrast, they may be confident with adults.
- Underachievement; homework/coursework may be of poor quality, not submitted on time or not handed in at all.
- Anxiety or concern over ill/disabled relative.
- Behavioural problems—there is often a big difference between the young person who seems 'mature beyond their years' in the home environment where they are very protective of a disabled relative, and the young person who takes out their pent-up frustration or stress at school.
- Physical problems such as back pain from lifting an adult (*see* www. youngcarers.net/i_care_for_someone_who/37/54).

What to do next

- Speak to the young person in private—do not confront them in front of their peers. Explain the confidentiality rules that you operate within in age-appropriate language.
- Establish what caring tasks they are performing and why. Find out how their caring role affects them: Are they being bullied? Do they struggle with schoolwork? Do they miss out on extra-curricular activities? Do they worry when they are out of contact with home? How can you help with these issues?
- With the young person's permission, speak to their parent/s and explain the effect that the young person's caring role is having on his or her education. Are there other forms of support open to the family or another family member that could help more? Remember—few parents choose a caring role for their child: it is often the only option they are aware of and many feel very guilty about the effect their illness or disability has on their child.
- Explain to parents and children that they may be entitled to an assessment of their needs from social services, who may be able to help them.
- Help the family to contact other agencies, or your nearest **Young Carers Project** if they want you to (*see* www.youngcarer.com/showPage.php?file=projects.htm).

Adapted from www.carers.org/professionals/young-carers

History of abuse

Studies have found that almost half of psychiatric inpatients have histories of physical and/or sexual abuse. Rates were higher for childhood mental health problems, personality disorders, anxiety and acute stress disorders, and major mood disorders.

Any adult who works with children or young people and suspects that a young person may be at risk or has been abused must share this information with an appropriate agency, e.g. social services. *See* Chapter 7 for further details on information sharing.

Emotional abuse

Emotional abuse tends not to be addressed with the same urgency as the physical abuse of children, but early intervention is necessary to avoid long-term consequences for the emotional health of the child.

For the purposes of child protection, the Department of Health uses the following definition of emotional abuse:

> '... the persistent emotional ill-treatment of a child such as to cause severe and persistent adverse effects on the child's emotional development. It may involve conveying to children that they are worthless or unloved, inadequate, or valued only insofar as they meet the needs of another person. It may feature age or developmentally inappropriate expectations being imposed on children. It may involve causing children frequently to feel frightened or in danger, or the exploitation or corruption of children. Some level of emotional abuse is involved in all types of ill treatment of a child, though it may occur alone.'

Research suggests that emotional abuse can be associated with parents who are alcoholic or abuse street drugs or other substances, with parents who have depression, in families where there is domestic violence, and among children with physical disabilities and their siblings.

As above, if you suspect that a child may be experiencing emotional abuse, please share the information with an appropriate agency.

Discrimination

Discrimination on the grounds of race, sex, sexuality and disability can induce fear, undermine self-confidence, and reduce opportunities in education, housing and employment—all of which can be distressing experiences for an adolescent.

For example, issues of sexual identity can be especially troubling during teenage years, when identity in general is being questioned. Young lesbians and gays are often told they are going through 'a phase', which they will grow out of. This can encourage denial and promote negative thoughts about being lesbian or gay.

People from minority ethnic groups are more likely than the general population to experience social exclusion, to be poor and live in deprived areas. Unemployment, low wages, long working hours, overcrowding and poor housing can all have an impact on children's psychological development.

Children from minority ethnic communities are vulnerable to the influences of racism and prejudice. Ideas, beliefs, feelings, attitudes and behaviour relating to race and skin colour are communicated by parents, siblings, peers, teachers, the media, churches and other cultural agents. This area is closely linked with bullying.

Refugees

Young refugees face a series of problems, including isolation and feelings of loss, confusion and sometimes bereavement. They may have witnessed extreme violence, which may cause disturbing memories and induce feelings of guilt about surviving. There may be conflicts within their families if their values conflict with the traditional attitudes of their parents or elders. They may have problems with their cultural identity as they begin to settle into a new society.

Many refugee families will also be facing the practical problems of surviving in the UK. Many refugees are housed in bed-and-breakfast accommodation in squalid conditions. Parents are under stress and find it difficult to cope with their children in these conditions. They may find it difficult to register with a general practitioner (GP) and they very often have no medical records.

Additional resources

For further information and support, visit:
www.refugeecouncil.org.uk

If you become aware that one of the young people you are working with is in this situation, link them into your local refugee advice centre through the website above.

Disability

Physical disability may affect communication skills and mobility, and it may limit access to both work and leisure activities. This may lead to the person with the disability feeling demoralised by a lack of opportunities and discriminatory attitudes, and this may have an impact on their mental health. People with a disability can also experience bullying.

Mental health and learning disabilities

Excellent information from the Royal College of Psychiatrists can be viewed as a PDF or ordered in leaflet form.
www.rcpsych.ac.uk/mentalhealthinformation/mentalhealthproblems/
depression/learningdisability.aspx

ALCOHOL AND DRUG USE

Alcohol

The World Health Organisation's European Charter on Alcohol, signed by all member states of the EU, states:

> 'All children and adolescents have the right to grow up in an environment protected from the negative consequences of alcohol consumption, and to the extent possible, from the promotion of alcoholic beverages.'

In the inter-war period, young people aged 18 to 24 were the lightest drinkers in the population, and the group most likely not to drink at all. By the 1980s, this group had become the heaviest drinkers in the population and the least likely to abstain. Nowadays, many young people drink regularly by the age of 14 or 15, and one survey found that more than a quarter of boys aged nine to 10 were drinking regularly at home. The latest survey data shows that girls are now binge drinking as much as boys. Minority ethnic teenagers are less likely to drink alcohol than their white counterparts.

Binge drinking can result in unsafe sex, injury and illness, dangerous behaviour, and is linked to trouble with the law.

In the long-term, continued alcohol misuse is likely to affect social functioning, including school performance. Alcohol misuse by young people is associated with heavy drinking in later life, and there is an association between alcohol and the use of illegal drugs. There is also evidence that alcohol misuse is associated with poor nutrition, and that alcohol can disrupt some of the biological mechanisms involved in physical growth during puberty. It may also impair psychological and emotional development. *See* further information in Chapter 6.

Drugs

The taking of legal and illegal drugs can be both physically and emotionally addictive, and should not be ignored as a passing phase. Use of illegal drugs such as cannabis and ecstasy has been linked with the development of depression and psychosis in some susceptible individuals. Some people also react to steroids, used to enhance performance in sport, by becoming violent or manic. There is the additional risk of hepatitis and HIV infection if drugs are injected.

See Chapter 6 for further information, advice and activities in relation to drugs and alcohol.

Additional resources

The Mind website gives a good background on factors that contribute to mental health problems in children and young people. www.mind.org.uk/help/people_groups_and_communities/children_young_people_and_mental_health

CONDITIONS

The three most common groups of childhood mental health issues are:
- emotional disorders (such as depression, anxiety and obsessions)
- hyperactivity (e.g. inattention and overactivity)
- conduct disorders (e.g. awkward, troublesome, aggressive and antisocial behaviour).

Less-common mental disorders include autistic spectrum disorders, neurological disorders such as Tourette's syndrome, and eating disorders.

We will consider here the most common mental health problems that we may come across. These are considered in brief to give basic insight into the conditions.

Depression

About two in 100 children under the age of 12 are depressed to the extent that they would benefit from seeing a specialist child psychiatrist. About 4 or 5% in this age group show significant distress and some of these could be described as on the edge of depression. The rate increases with age, so that at least 5% of teenagers are seriously depressed and at least twice that number show significant distress. These figures apply to children living in stable, settled populations in reasonably good social circumstances. In troubled, inner city areas with high rates of broken homes, poor community support and raised neighbourhood crime rates, the level of depression may be double.

Causes of depression amongst children and young people are as many and varied as in the adult population, and can be linked to family or relationship problems, academic pressure or worries about the future.

Symptoms of depression

The symptoms listed below are common indicators of depression. If a child or young person has some of these symptoms for most of the day, for more days than not, and if there is significant impact on daily functioning, he or she may be depressed:

- feeling sad, miserable, tearful—persistent low mood that does not lift
- irritability—persistent oversensitivity, which can appear as aggressive outbursts
- social withdrawal—isolation from friends and family, hiding away
- poor concentration—difficulty with attention, decision-making and memory
- altered sleep pattern—difficulty in going off to sleep; disturbed sleep
- altered appetite/weight—loss or gain in appetite and weight
- low self-esteem—low opinion of self, one's own attributes and capabilities
- anhedonia—loss of pleasure in hobbies, work or relationships
- hopelessness/helplessness—pervasive negative thinking style
- suicidal thoughts—thoughts that life is not worth living
- self-blame/guilt—excessive preoccupation with past actions.

This information is from the teacher training pack 'Depression in Young People', produced by the Young People's Unit at the Royal Edinburgh Hospital.

Thinking about depression

Have a brief discussion about depression. State that there are varying degrees of depression, ranging from times when you feel 'down' or 'sad', all the way to clinical depression.

Continuum

Draw a straight line on the board. Put 'feeling down or sad' at the left end and 'clinical depression' on the right end. Explain that all of us will experience some degree of depression, e.g. when someone dies, significant losses/changes occur, relationships break up, etc. Give an example when you might have felt depressed. Put an **'X'** on the continuum where you felt it would be. The more symptoms of depression and the length of time you experience it will all help determine where it would be on the continuum. Stress that the closer to the right end, the more important it is to get help. Clinical depression needs professional help.

Brainstorm

Brainstorm events or periods of time when the students have felt depressed. It can be their own experiences or those of others. List them on the board when completed.

Have the group quietly think back to an event or time period in their life when they felt really sad or down.

List words he/she felt when this event happened, like lonely, unhappy, angry, etc. List the feeling words. Affirm all answers.

Ask: 'How did you act differently when you were sad?' You might start with, 'You wanted to be alone', etc. List responses.

Ask: 'What thoughts went through your mind when you were sad?' You could start with: 'Why does this happen?' List responses.

Discuss with the young people the reason we did this activity. Regardless of the event, our answers were very similar. We all feel very much the same when we go through these events. Unless this event was quite recent, most of us don't feel that way anymore. Ask young people if they still feel the way they listed. Most will not. We all experience times when we're depressed. When we are depressed, we don't feel the way we normally do, we don't act the way we normally do, and we don't think the way we normally do. However, we all feel differently now than we did when we experienced these sad life events.

Have the young people mentally recall their event again. Ask if they remember anyone saying something to them when they were sad that made them feel better. List responses. Conclude with the most important things we can do when others/we are depressed: TALK, LISTEN, and GET HELP.

Highlight that when clinically depressed, however, people can't pull themselves out of it. This can be a serious health problem that can affect the ability to carry on daily life. When the feelings of sadness, hopelessness or despair last longer than a few weeks and interfere with interests and activities, professional help is needed. Professionals can give counselling and medication to help those who are clinically depressed get back to feeling normal again.

Self-harm

Self-harm includes a range of behaviours such as self-cutting, burning and deliberately ingesting harmful substances. Although acts of self-harm may be suicidal in intent or associated with suicidal thoughts, there may be other motivations.

The person who self-harms may be trying to take control of distress, express painful feelings or may use their destructive behaviour as a form of release.

Research suggests self-harm is becoming increasingly common among young people. Self-harm is more common in adolescents who have been bullied and is strongly associated with physical and sexual abuse in both boys and girls. It is also associated with anxiety about sexual orientation.

Why do people harm themselves?

The underlying reasons why a person might self-harm are often complex and may be difficult to understand. It usually stems from the difficulties that people are experiencing within themselves. Different people self-harm for different reasons at different times.

There are some common misconceptions concerning self-harm:

- self-harm is not attention-seeking behaviour; in fact, most people try to hide their injuries
- self-harm is not a failed attempt at suicide; on the contrary—many people who self-harm see it as a way of staying alive
- self-harm is not manipulative behaviour: many people who self-harm are often unaware of the effect that their self-harming has on others.

How to help someone who appears to be self-harming

- Pay attention to the person's injuries; by doing this you affirm that the person and his body are worth caring about.
- Don't just focus on the injuries. It's important that you appreciate how difficult your friend or relative is finding life. Showing the person that you want to understand will matter a great deal.
- Begin by gently encouraging your friend to examine his feelings and to talk to someone about why he self-harms. You may find what he has to say difficult to hear. If it feels too much for you, help your friend to find someone else to talk to.
- Encourage the person to seek advice from his doctor or nurse.
- Keep emphasising all the non-harming aspects of the person's life to help develop and support his sense of self-worth.
- Don't expect change to happen quickly.

Source: www.mind.org.uk/help/diagnoses_and_conditions/self-harm#help

Suicide

Some people have a very strong, clear desire for death. They may feel hopeless about the future, believing that things will never get better. Suicide may seem to be the only way of solving problems, once and for all, and ending the emotional pain of living. However, a lot of self-destructive emotion, thought and behaviour is far more confused than this. Someone who feels that their situation and problems have become intolerable may see no alternative but to attempt to kill himself. Yet, this person is likely to have extremely mixed feelings about this, and feel very afraid.

Additional resources

See the 'Mind' website for information on how to help someone who is suicidal:

www.mind.org.uk/help/medical_and_alternative_care/how_to_help_someone_who_is_suicidal

> 'Only when you know what it is like to feel depressed, to feel you are dying inside, can you know what it is like to be suicidal, to think that the whole dreadful, terrible, nagging, awful pain of it all might be swept away by a simple, single act of self destruction.'
>
> – Spike Milligan

A study of life events preceding suicide suggests that reasons given fall into four categories—relationship problems, illness, family disruption and loss. These broad categories cover a wide range of individual stories, for example, sexuality, arguing with parents, wanting to be with someone who has died, being diagnosed HIV-positive, failing an exam. (*See* the fact sheets on children and young people's mental health at www.mind.org.uk to learn more.)

At-risk groups

- Race and cultural background can be a major influence on suicidal behaviour. For example, one study of young people of Asian origin in the UK found that the suicide rate of 16 to 24-year-old women was three times higher than that of white women in the same age range. Asian women's groups have linked these high suicide rates to cultural pressures: conservative parental values and traditions such as arranged marriages may clash with the wishes and expectations of young women themselves.
- People with serious mental health problems such as bipolar disorder (manic depression) or schizophrenia have a considerably higher chance of dying by suicide than the general population.

- Misuse of alcohol and drugs increases the risk of suicide, especially in young men.
- Attempted suicide is much higher amongst the unemployed than amongst people who are in work. This is also true of homeless people. Young gay men and lesbians are particularly at risk too, possibly because of the discrimination they face in our society.
- A history of physical or sexual abuse puts young people at increased risk of suicide or deliberate self-harm. A violent home life is also likely to contribute.
- Relationship problems, especially disturbed family relationships, are often in the background when someone attempts suicide.
- Men are more likely to take their own lives than women.
- If someone has a long-standing or painful physical problem, they may become depressed, and this in turn makes them more prone to suicidal feelings.
- The suicide rate for men in prison is five times the total male suicide rate.

What are the warning signs of suicide?

- Feelings of failure, loss of self-esteem, isolation and hopelessness.
- Sleep problems, particularly waking up early.
- A sense of uselessness and futility. Feeling 'What's the point?'
- Taking less care of themselves; for example, eating badly or not caring what they look like.
- Suddenly making out a will or taking out life insurance.
- Talking about suicide. It's a myth that people who talk about suicide don't go through with it. In fact, most people who have taken their own lives have spoken about it to someone.
- A marked change of behaviour. Someone may appear to be calm and at peace for the first time or, more usually, may be withdrawn and have difficulty communicating.
- There is a particular risk of suicide when someone who has been suffering from depression is just beginning to recover. They may have the energy to commit suicide that they lacked when they were severely depressed.

How can you help?

- It's important to encourage the person to talk about his or her despairing feelings.
- Don't dismiss expressions of hopelessness as a 'cry for help' or try to jolly them out of it. Talking openly about the possibility of suicide will not make it more likely to happen. Just being there for the person and listening in an accepting way can help him or her feel less isolated and frightened.
- It may be useful to emphasise to the suicidal person that suicide may not be the quick answer he or she is hoping for. Indeed, an attempt may fail and result in greater suffering, such as severe disablement or brain damage.
- It's important to persuade someone who is feeling suicidal to get some outside support. The person's GP is a good starting-point. He or she can arrange for the person to get professional help, such as psychotherapy or counselling, and may prescribe antidepressants, if appropriate.
- There are organisations, such as the Samaritans, that offer emergency helplines for people who are feeling desperate. They may also offer ongoing support in the form of self-help groups, general advice and information.
- It's a good idea to discuss strategies for seeking help if the person has suicidal thoughts. Creating a personal support list is a useful way of reviewing every conceivable option. The list may include the names, phone numbers and addresses of individuals, helplines, organisations and professionals available for support. Persuade the person to keep this list by the phone and to agree to call someone when they are feeling suicidal.

Important contacts

Papyrus (Prevention of Young Suicide) *Committed to the prevention of young suicide*
Helpline: 0800 068 41 41
Web: www.papyrus-uk.org

Samaritans
24-hour emotional support
Helpline: 08457 90 90 90
Email: jo@samaritans.org
Web: www.samaritans.org

Eating distress

Many children and young people struggle with their body image. They are, after all, growing up in a culture where they are constantly faced with images and messages about the desirability of being thin from television, magazines and advertisements.

Eating distress can take different forms. People with anorexia starve themselves by eating little or nothing, while people with bulimia binge on food, then induce vomiting and/or take laxatives. Both conditions can cause severe weight loss or gain, other physical health problems and can sometimes result in death. Between one in five to one in seven of those with anorexia die as a result of their illness or take their own lives. The average age of anorexia onset is 15 and the average age of bulimia onset is 18.

Eating problems are more common among girls and young women, but more boys and young men are experiencing problems with food. Around 10% of anorexia cases occur in males. In the past, there has been less cultural pressure on men than women to stay slim, but this is changing. *See* Chapter 2 for more information, advice and activities regarding eating disorders.

Attention deficit hyperactivity disorder (ADHD)

Some children are consistently difficult to manage. They may have problems concentrating, be quick to react, tend to act impulsively, be unable to settle, lack self-confidence and be both disruptive and destructive. These children are often described as suffering from 'attention deficit hyperactivity disorder' (ADHD).

Some child psychiatrists advocate treatment with amphetamine-related stimulant drugs such as Ritalin (methylphenidate). *The British National Formulary* advises that this drug not be given to children under six, and cautions that it should be used selectively, since one side effect is to slow growth, and the long-term effects are not known. Many experts believe that drug treatment is only appropriate in the most severe cases, and would advocate its use only in combination with psychological therapies.

It has been suggested that ADHD is closely related to lack of sleep. Many parents do not put their children to bed nearly as early as was normal 30 or 40 years ago, and many children have television and computers in their bedrooms, encouraging them to stay awake. Lack of sleep causes people to feel restless and makes concentration difficult. Diet is also implicated in ADHD. Children's behaviour and concentration frequently improves with a diet that is low in sugar, carbonated drinks and artificial colourants.

COMBATING MENTAL HEALTH ISSUES

Resilience

A resilient person is one who exhibits positive adaptation in circumstances where one might expect, due to unusual levels of stress, difficulty in coping.

Research has shown that the most powerful resilience-promoting factors for young people are a supportive family and peer support. Resilience can only be developed through exposure to stressors. Having to deal with challenging situations will enable children to develop emotional and physical confidence. However, the presence of one risk factor increases the likelihood that other risk factors will be present.

Risk factors heighten the probability that children will experience poor outcomes. Resilience factors increase the likelihood that children will resist or recover from exposure to adversities. Positive child development is not simply a matter of reducing or eliminating risk factors and promoting resilience. The successful management of risk is a powerful resilience-promoting factor in itself. However, risk factors are cumulative. Children may often be able to overcome and even learn from single or moderate risks, but when risk factors accumulate, children's capacity to cope rapidly diminishes. Resilience factors operate in three dimensions: the individual, the family and the external environment.

Resilience factors

The child	The family	The environment
Temperament (active, good-natured)	Warm, supportive parents	Supportive extended family
Female prior to adolescence and male during adolescence	Good parent-child relationships	Successful school experiences
Age (Younger children tend to be more resilient)	Parental harmony	Friendship networks
Higher IQ	Valued social role, e.g. care of siblings	Valued social role, e.g. a job, volunteering, helping neighbours
Social skills	Close relationship with one parent	Close relationship with unrelated mentor
Personal awareness		Member of a religion or faith community
Feelings of empathy		
Internal locus of control		
Humour		
Attractiveness		

As can be seen, some of these factors are partly biogenetic, and their sensitivity to change or manipulation is limited. Most, however, are familiar variables and present a wide range of possibilities for positive change—but there is no simple association between stress and gain. Some stressors may trigger resilient assets in children, others may compound difficulties. If children are subjected to a relentless stream of multiple adversities, negative consequences are highly likely to follow.

We can see from this brief summary that resilience-promoting factors remain fairly consistent, with supportive families, positive peer relationships, external networks and the opportunity to develop self-esteem and efficacy through valued social roles being of particular importance.

TREATMENTS

When we think about treatments, we tend to immediately think about therapy and medication; this is because we come from a society that has traditionally valued the medical model. However, we mustn't forget non-medical strategies that can enhance emotional well-being, such as sports activities, dance, group activities that explore working together, and a healthy diet.

 Can you incorporate fun activities into the group's schedule, e.g. hosting 'make your own pizza' night or a street dance session?

The following outlines the traditional therapies that are offered to people with diagnosable mental health issues.

Talking treatments

Counselling and psychotherapy are talking treatments used by trained counsellors or psychotherapists to help people with their emotional problems. Both offer the individual, family or group a space to talk about their problems, to explore the past and possibly to find causes and possible solutions.

Medication

Medical consensus seems to be that doctors should prescribe psychiatric drugs to children and young people sparingly and in conjunction with talking treatments.

In general, how can we support young people's emotional health?

We are likely to be involved with young people on a sessional basis and hence cannot provide any intense interventions for young people who are experiencing emotional difficulties. However, I have included some information and activities here that can be explored on a sessional basis either with groups or one to one. It should be stressed that where there is an identified issue, it is always good practice to liaise with other professionals involved in the young person's care, e.g. the GP, teacher, social worker, etc., so there is a team approach to a young person's welfare. This is for your benefit as well as the young person's.

 Do a session with your young people on positive self-talk using the guidance below.

Display the guidance on positive self-talk where young people can refer to it, or supply the information in handout format.

 Invite a yoga teacher to come and do some simple relaxation techniques with your group.

 If you feel confident, put on some soft music, darken the room and take your group through the three relaxation steps below— breathing, muscle relaxation and visualisation.

 Display a 'building confidence and self-esteem' poster for your young people to see, or make it available as a handout—or do a short session on the techniques described on the poster.

 Encourage your young people to volunteer and hence improve their self-esteem by contributing to society. The group could volunteer to pick up litter, make cakes for the elderly, etc.

Positive self-talk

Self-talk is the talking you do in your own head about yourself and the things that happen, your own 'running commentary' on your life. Often this self-talk happens so automatically that you are barely aware of it. However, what you say to yourself can have a big effect on the way that you feel, and on what you can achieve. Your self-talk can be like an internal coach, encouraging you, boosting your confidence, believing in you, and motivating you to achieve your goals, or it can be like an internal bully, undermining you, criticising you and oppressing you when you're down.

Sports psychologists have long recognised the importance of positive self-talk in helping athletes achieve their potential. Everyone who plays competitive sport or who competes at a serious level faces adversity and obstacles to success: physical pain, poor conditions, strong opponents, fatigue. The only way an athlete can succeed in the face of these difficulties is to have powerful self-belief and great determination. Positive self-talk is one tool that athletes use to achieve their best in competition.

Changing your self-talk

There are three steps to changing your self-talk so it works for you rather than against you:

1 **Identify your self-talk.** Self-talk is often so habitual that people are unaware that they are doing it at all. If you are going to change your self-talk, you need to be aware of these thoughts as they happen. Take some time to notice the things you say to yourself during your day.

2 **Assess your self-talk.** Is it negative or positive? If it is negative, ask yourself these questions:
   - is there any evidence for this thought?
   - is there any evidence against it?
   - is this the way I would talk to a friend who was in my position?
   - are there any more positive ways of viewing this situation?
   - am I keeping things in perspective?
   - even if there is some validity to this thought, is it useful spending my energy thinking about it?

3 **Change your self-talk.** If you decide that your self-talk is unhelpful or wrong, replace the negative thoughts with a more positive alternative.

Changing self-talk requires some time and practice, since our ways of thinking tend to be quite ingrained. You will probably need to keep working on the three-step process above for some time before it becomes second nature.

Relaxation

Relaxation is a great technique for improving your mental health. Although it is good to use relaxation techniques when you are stressed, it is even better to include some relaxation in your everyday routine. Relaxation can help you to cope with stressful situations.

Breathing techniques

There are many breathing techniques that can be used to help create a feeling of relaxation. When feeling stressed or anxious, it can help to take just 10 slow, deep breaths, breathing in through the nose and out through the mouth. If you have the time and the privacy, you can sit or lie down and close your eyes, then focus your attention on your breathing. Inhale slowly to the bottom of your lungs, hold the air for a few seconds, then slowly exhale. Continue this pattern of breathing for a while, and you will notice that you start to feel peaceful and calm.

Progressive muscle relaxation

This technique involves progressively tensing and then relaxing all the different muscle groups in your body. Start with your toes and feet, tightening the muscles as much as you can without discomfort. Hold the tension for a count of five, then allow the muscles to completely relax. Now move to your lower legs and repeat the process. Continue up the body, all the way to your face and scalp, until your whole body is relaxed.

Visualisation

Sit or lie down somewhere comfortable and quiet and close your eyes. You might like to listen to some music as you do this, but if you do you should choose gentle music without words. Think of a beautiful, relaxing setting somewhere in nature. It might be somewhere you typically feel peaceful and relaxed, or it might be a made-up place. For example, you could try to think about a beach with soft sand, the waves rolling in, the sun going down, and that you are lying down with the wind moving through your hair. Try to use all your senses to make the scene come alive. Feel the sand running through your fingers, hear the soothing sound of the surf. Smell the salty breeze. Stay in this place for as long as you need to feel peaceful and relaxed.

Additional resources

For further information on relaxation techniques, visit: www.embracethefuture.org.au/youth/relaxation.aspx

Building confidence and self-esteem

Self-esteem is what you think about yourself as a person and how good you feel about yourself.

Strategies for raising self-esteem:
- be positive
- take notice when you are negative towards yourself and try to stop the negative thinking
- remember the good things. Write them down
- think big, but be realistic
- try new things
- think about your qualities that have helped you in life. Make a list and think about how you might use these qualities in the future
- get involved. Participate
- do things that you love doing and you know you are good at
- let yourself make mistakes. Learn from your mistakes
- try to believe in yourself
- try positive affirmations. Positive affirmations are positive comments or statements that you can keep telling yourself (either out loud or in your head).

Examples of positive affirmations:
- i can do it!
- i will get the assignment done by the due date!
- i am clever!
- we can win!
- i can get a part-time job!

Sometimes trying to be positive can be very hard. Often when something goes wrong it is easy to believe that 'everything always happens to me'. This is negative self-talk. To check on your self-talk, you could ask:
- am I focusing on the negative things—have I forgotten about what I can actually do?
- are things as bad as they seem?
- am I being negative?
- am I being realistic?
- how can I be more positive?

Getting involved

Being involved in your community helps you to be more resilient. When you are involved with others, particularly in activities that are meaningful, your self-esteem grows and you have a greater sense of purpose. It also helps because you tend to develop connections with other people who can act as supports, and you feel that you belong to a group.

Being involved in activities with a meaningful social purpose can be particularly good. Some examples might be:
- volunteering your time for a charity that supports a cause you believe in (for example, protecting the environment)
- getting involved in school working groups and committees
- being involved in political change, e.g. peacefully demonstrating against a law you think is wrong
- taking part in community activities like tree-planting days.

These examples are all activities that have a clear social benefit. These types of activities are particularly good at promoting resiliency. But even participation in things like sporting groups or other recreational activities can help build resilience by helping to create connections with others, and help develop social and other skills. Some examples might be:
- taking part in a theatre production
- joining the local cricket or netball club
- playing in a band
- taking art, dance or martial arts classes.

Additional resources

Youth volunteer websites
www.vinspired.com
www.youthactionnetwork.org.uk

CHAPTER 4

Healthy eating

We are hearing more and more about the effects of eating habits on our future health. Heart disease and diabetes rates are rising, and obesity is increasingly prevalent. It is important to eat healthily at all ages; however, adolescence can be a time where eating habits can become erratic. This is due to a combination of factors, such as becoming increasingly independent of parents, starting to make one's own choices regarding food, the increasing influence of peers and a raised awareness of body image, which can lead to fad diets.

This chapter will look at what the nutritional requirements are for adolescence, what the eating habits of young people are, and will also examine what healthy eating is for a young person. We will look more closely at certain areas such as obesity, dieting, vegetarianism, and sport, work through how to calculate body mass index (BMI) and include a few suggestions for activities and recipes that emphasise healthy eating principles.

What is 'healthy eating'?

Good eating habits are generally acquired when young and persist throughout life. Eating foods in the proportions illustrated in the Balance of Good Health will help ensure children and teenagers obtain all the nutrients they require. A pictorial description of the Balance of Good Health is available from the following website: www.food.gov.uk/multimedia/pdfs/bghbooklet.pdf

The Balance of Good Health aims to give people a practical message about healthy eating. It is hoped that it will reduce the confusion about what healthy eating really means. It is based on the Government's Eight Guidelines for a Healthy Diet:

- enjoy your food
- eat a variety of different foods
- eat the right amount to be a healthy weight
- eat plenty of foods rich in starch and fibre

- eat plenty of fruits and vegetables
- don't eat too many foods that contain a lot of fat
- don't have sugary foods and drinks too often
- drink alcohol sensibly.

A healthy diet should also be based on as wide a variety of foods as possible, with the emphasis on foods of high nutrient density rather than those providing mainly energy and few nutrients, e.g. sweets, biscuits, crisps and fizzy drinks. The following table shows the recommended number of servings per day from each of the five food groups, the size of which will vary depending on appetite.

Food group	Suggested number of servings
Bread, cereals and potatoes	Foods from this group should form the basis of each meal
Fruits and vegetables	At least five
Milk and dairy foods, e.g. cheese and yogurt	At least three
Meat, poultry, fish and alternatives, e.g. eggs, pulses and nuts	Two
Foods containing fat and sugar, e.g. crisps, confectionery biscuits	Foods from this group should be eaten only occasionally, and in small amounts

Three main meals a day should be encouraged, with between-meal snacks as needed. These meals should consist of the healthier choices such as sandwiches or toast (preferably wholemeal), yogurt, fresh fruit and milk. Skipping meals can lead to reduced nutrient intakes, particularly if snacks that are high in fat and sugar but lack essential nutrients are taken instead. Foods such as chocolate, sweets, biscuits, cakes, crisps and sugary drinks should be consumed in moderation to help prevent obesity and tooth decay.

Breakfast, the most important meal of the day...

It is particularly important to have breakfast. Studies have shown that young people who eat breakfast have a better intake of vitamins and minerals than those who do not. In addition, breakfast improves the ability to concentrate and means you are less likely to snack on high-fat/high-sugar foods later in the morning. You don't need to have a cooked breakfast; a bowl of whole-grain breakfast cereal with milk and/or toast and a glass of fruit juice is fine. Recent studies have reported that around one in 10 primary school children skip breakfast. However, this number increases as children get older, particularly among girls.

Ask the young people to record what they eat for breakfast each day for a week. They should record their performance, endurance, and attitude during that week and discuss this information as a group. Is there a link between eating a nutritious breakfast and the levels of energy they feel and their ability to perform?

Divide the young people into small groups. Each group should plan two non-traditional breakfasts that would be nutritious, easy to prepare, and desirable to someone in the group's age. Have each group share their ideas.

The Balance of Good Health food guide

Starchy foods

Starchy foods such as bread, cereals, potatoes and pasta are a crucial part of a healthy diet. They contain carbohydrates, which are an essential source of energy. Starchy foods are fuel for your body. In a healthy meal, starchy foods should make up around a third of everything we eat. That means we should base our meals on these foods.

Try to choose wholegrain or wholemeal varieties, such as brown rice, wholewheat pasta and brown wholemeal bread. These contain more fibre (also called 'roughage') and usually more vitamins and minerals than white flour or white rice. There is also starch in beans, lentils, and peas.

Most of us need to include more starchy foods in our diets. Try having more wholewheat pasta or brown rice with your meal, and less sauce. Choose wholegrain cereals or porridge for breakfast.

Fibre

Fibre is the structural part of a plant that cannot be broken down by enzymes in digestion. Fibre is found in plant foods including fruits, vegetables, cereals, grains, nuts and legumes (dried peas, beans and lentils). Animal foods and dairy products do not contain fibre.

There are two main types of dietary fibre—soluble and insoluble fibre:

- **soluble fibre** may help to lower blood cholesterol levels when eaten as part of a well-balanced, low-fat diet. Soluble fibre may also assist in controlling blood sugar levels and in the treatment of obesity. Foods rich in soluble fibre include oats, fruit and vegetables.

- **insoluble fibre** helps prevent constipation. Foods rich in this type of fibre include wheat-based bread and cereals, vegetables, lentils and pasta.

The following are a few ways to incorporate fibre into your everyday diet:
- opt for wholegrain and wholemeal
- choose wholemeal breakfast cereals including bran cereals, muesli or rolled oats, such as porridge
- combine meat dishes with rice, beans, oatmeal and lentils
- eat all types of fruit and vegetables (fresh, dried, tinned) and where possible, also eat the skins on foods such as jacket potatoes.

Water

Next to oxygen, water is the human body's most important nutrient. Yet often we do not drink enough water to keep hydrated.

Water is part of the body's cells, tissues, organs and also every process in the body. In fact, up to 60% of the human body is water. Water is important for the following body functions:
- regulating body temperature
- removing waste from the body
- carrying nutrients, oxygen and glucose to the cells to give the body energy
- providing natural moisture to the skin and other tissues
- cushioning joints and helping to strengthen muscles
- keeping poo softer.

It is good to drink six to eight glasses of water a day.

Fruit and vegetables

Fruit and vegetables are a vital source of vitamins and minerals, and it is advised that we eat five portions of them a day. There is good evidence that people who eat five portions a day are at lower risk of coronary heart disease, stroke and certain cancers.

Eating five portions is not as hard as it might sound. Just one apple, banana, pear or similar sized fruit is one portion. A slice of pineapple or melon is one portion, and three heaped tablespoons of vegetables is another. A glass of fruit juice also counts as one portion (but more than one cannot be counted towards your five a day).

Having a sliced banana with your morning cereal is a quick way to get one portion. Have a tangerine mid-morning, and add a side salad to your lunch. Add a portion of vegetables to dinner, and snack on dried fruit in the evening to help you reach your five a day.

Vitamins

Vitamin A—Helps your eyes to see, especially at night; helps you see colours, grow in height, and maintain clear skin. Eat eggs, milk, carrots, apricots, nectarines and other yellow fruits, sweet potatoes and green leafy vegetables like spinach, liver.

Vitamin Bs—These vitamins help build nerves, make the heart work properly, make blood cells grow and make skin, nails and hair.

Foods you need to eat to get Vitamin Bs:
- B1 is in rice, peanuts, pork, liver, milk, yeast, wholemeal bread
- B2 is in milk, cheese, fish, leafy vegetables, liver
- B6 is in fish, bananas, chicken, pork, whole grains, beans
- B12 is in fish, beef, pork, milk, cheese, liver
- folic acid is in avocados, carrots, egg yolks, pumpkins, orange and grapefruit juices, liver, beans.

Vitamin C—Maintains gums, skin, muscles. Helps cuts and wounds heal and helps the body resist some bacterial and viral infections. Eat fresh fruits like oranges, lemons, kiwis, strawberries, raspberries, and black and blueberries. Also eat tomatoes, broccoli, potatoes, spinach and other green leafy vegetables.

Vitamin D—Helps make bones and teeth strong. It is not only present in lots of foods, but is also made in the skin in response to sunlight. Eat fish such as salmon, tuna and sardines, plus milk and cod liver oil.

Vitamin E—Helps make red blood cells, muscles and other tissues. It also helps fight some of the poisons that the body might be exposed to. Eat nuts, soya beans, leafy green vegetables such as broccoli, sprouts and spinach, and eggs, seafood and oils.

Vitamin K—Helps the blood clot. Eat leafy green vegetables, liver, pork, milk and yogurt.

Minerals

Minerals are essential nutrients that the body needs in small amounts to work properly. We need them in the form they are found in food. Minerals can be found in varying amounts in a variety of foods such as meat, cereals (including cereal products such as bread), fish, milk and dairy foods, vegetables, fruit (especially dried fruit) and nuts.

Minerals are necessary for three main reasons:
- to build strong bones and teeth
- to control body fluids inside and outside cells
- to turn the food we eat into energy.

These are all essential minerals: calcium, iron, magnesium, phosphorus, potassium, sodium and sulphur.

Trace elements

Trace elements are also essential nutrients that your body needs to work properly, but in much smaller amounts than vitamins and minerals.

Trace elements are found in small amounts in a variety of foods such as meat, fish, cereals, milk and dairy foods, vegetables and nuts.

These are all trace elements: boron, cobalt, copper, chromium, fluoride, iodine, manganese, molybdenum, selenium, silicon and zinc.

Meat, fish, eggs and beans

These foods are all sources of protein, which is essential for growth and repair of the body. Meat is a good source of protein, and so are the vitamins and minerals such as iron, zinc and B vitamins. Meat is also one of the main sources of vitamin B12. Try to eat lean cuts of meat whenever possible to cut down on fat, and make sure you always cook meat thoroughly.

Fish is another important source of protein. There is evidence that people who eat two portions or more a week of oily fish such as sardines, mackerel, herring and salmon are at lower risk of heart disease. That's because oily fish contain high levels of a 'good fat' called omega-3.

Eggs and pulses—including beans, nuts and seeds—are also great sources of protein. But eggs and some nuts contain high levels of fat, so eat them in moderation.

Milk and dairy foods

Milk and dairy foods such as cheese and yogurt are also sources of protein. They contain calcium, which helps keep bones healthy. But some dairy products have a high saturated fat content, and eating too much saturated fat is linked to heart disease. To enjoy the health benefits of dairy without eating too much fat, try using skimmed milk, low-fat hard cheeses or cottage cheese, and low-fat yogurt instead of cream or soured cream.

Fat and sugar

Of all the five food groups, it is our consumption of foods that are high in fat and sugar that does the most to make our diet unbalanced. Fats and sugar are powerful sources of energy for the body. But when we eat too much of them we consume more energy than we burn, meaning we put on weight. Obesity—linked to diabetes, heart disease, stroke and certain cancers—can be the result.

Saturated fat, contained in high levels in such foods as pies, meat products, sausages, cakes and biscuits, can raise your cholesterol level, and increase your risk of heart disease.

Unsaturated fat, on the other hand, can lower cholesterol and provide the essential fatty acids needed to stay healthy. Oily fish, nuts and seeds, avocados, olive oils and vegetable oils are sources of unsaturated fat.

There are two kinds of food containing sugar, too. Sugar occurs naturally in foods such as fruit and milk. But sugar is added to processed foods such as fizzy drinks, cakes, biscuits, chocolate, pastries, ice cream and jam. It's also contained in some ready-made savoury foods such as pasta sauces and baked beans.

It's the foods with added sugar that most of us need to cut down on. Instead of a fizzy drink, have a half-and-half mixture of fruit juice and water. Make a pasta sauce yourself instead of buying it ready-made. Have dried fruit for a snack instead of a chocolate bar.

Nutritional requirements in adolescence

Young people's diets should sustain growth, promote both current and future health, and be enjoyable. During adolescence a number of physiological changes occur. These include a marked increase in growth (the pubertal growth spurt) and considerable gains in bone and muscle. These changes influence nutritional requirements and demand for both nutrients and energy are high. This makes teenagers particularly vulnerable to deficiency. Anything that increases nutritional needs, such as participation in competitive sport, or interferes with intake, such as dieting, also increases the risk of dietary inadequacy.

SPECIFIC NUTRIENTS REQUIRED FOR A TEENAGE DIET

Iron

Iron requirements are markedly increased during adolescence. For both boys and girls, extra iron is needed due to increases in lean body mass, blood volume and haemoglobin. In addition, girls need to replace the iron lost with menstruation. This, together with low dietary iron intake, can make teenage girls particularly vulnerable to iron deficiency anaemia.

Young people should eat whole grains rich in iron like cereals, breads, rice and pasta; green vegetables like spinach, kale and broccoli; eggs; red meats like pork, lamb and beef; dark meat poultry; and beans which are rich in nutrients like lentils, black beans, chick peas and dried fruits.

Calcium

During childhood and adolescence, there is a once-in-a-lifetime opportunity to build strong bones. About 90% of the total body mineral density is achieved by 17 years of age. At the peak of the growth spurt a large amount of calcium is retained.

The most recent national dietary survey of children and adolescents reported that one in four older girls (11 to 18 years) had calcium intakes below the recommended nutrient intake. Inadequate intake of calcium during adolescence may result in failure to reach peak bone mass. This, in turn, may increase the risk of developing osteoporosis in later life. **Eat:** milk, cheese and yogurt.

Other minerals

Requirements for magnesium, phosphorus and iodine are known to be high due to the muscular and skeletal development that takes place during adolescence. Zinc is also an essential mineral for growth and sexual development. **Eat:** a wide range of vegetables, wholegrains and nuts.

Vitamins

Adolescents require quite large amounts of the B vitamins thiamin, riboflavin and niacin, in line with the increased requirement for energy. Folate requirements are also likely to be high at this time because of the involvement of folate in DNA and RNA synthesis in cell growth. **Eat:** a range of fruits and vegetables.

WHAT ARE TEENAGERS EATING?

In 2000, the government published the National Diet and Nutrition Survey of Young People, which reported on the eating habits of 4- to 18-year-olds in the UK. The survey revealed:

- the most commonly eaten foods were white bread, savoury snacks, biscuits, potatoes (including chips) and chocolate
- fizzy drinks were the most popular drink
- most young people drank milk, but the proportion not drinking milk increased with age
- chicken and turkey were the most commonly eaten meats
- on average, children ate less than half the recommended five portions of fruit and vegetables per day
- one in five children ate no fruit at all during the week of the study
- one in five young people took vitamin and mineral supplements

- ten per cent of older girls (15 to 18 year olds) said they were vegetarian
- sixteen per cent of the older girls were on a diet (compared to only 3% of 15- to 18-year-old boys)
- the majority of children could be classed as inactive: 40% of boys and 60% of girls did less than one hour of moderate physical activity per day
- the majority of children had adequate intakes of most nutrients and there was no evidence of widespread malnourishment
- in older age groups (15 to 18 years old), intakes of some minerals were lower than recommended
- zinc, potassium, magnesium, calcium, iron, iodine and copper were all low in older girls. A low intake of milk and red meat is likely to contribute to the poor intake of many of these nutrients
- analysis of blood samples found poor nutritional status with regard to iron and some B vitamins
- a large number of children also had low blood levels of vitamin D, which is important for calcium absorption and therefore bone health
- the intake of saturated fats, non-milk sugars and salt were all higher than recommended, and fibre intake was well below the adult recommendation.

Encourage young people to keep a food diary; it can help identify any overindulgence in certain types of food. As well as noting what they eat, they should also note down the time, place and how they feel. Mood often plays a big part in what and how much you eat. Understanding what makes you want to eat more can help break bad eating habits.

TEENAGE EATING HABITS

There are many factors that affect eating behaviour in adolescence. These include:

- physiological needs and characteristics
- health
- family unit and family characteristics
- peer pressure
- social and cultural norms and values
- media influences such as advertising
- available income
- personal values and beliefs
- nutrition knowledge
- body image.

Independence

Adolescence is a time of increasing independence. Changing lifestyles, social values and spending power have contributed to an increased reliance on snacks and 'fast foods' in teenagers. Regular meals are often replaced by grazing throughout the day. While the grazing pattern of eating can be healthy provided it is part of a balanced diet, in practice it often results in a diet that is too high in fat and sugar and low in other essential nutrients.

Fast food

The lower fat options for 'fast foods' such as wholemeal bread sandwiches, jacket potato and filling and grilled burgers should usually be chosen in preference to chips and fried fish or burgers. Choosing thick cut chips rather than French fries can also reduce the fat content of a fast food meal, and the addition of salad will improve the overall balance.

Skipping meals

Skipping meals, particularly breakfast, also becomes increasingly common as children get older. As previously discussed, studies have shown that as many as one in five teenage girls miss breakfast, with consequences for both nutritional intake and cognition.

Changes that can lead to a healthier diet for adolescents include:

- eating more fruit and vegetables
- replacing crisps, cakes, pastries, sweets and biscuits with more bread (preferably wholemeal) and bread products such as teacakes, fruit buns, crumpets, plain muffins and bread sticks
- reducing consumption of soft drinks such as fizzy drinks and squash, which are high in sugar
- drinking more milk
- using leaner meat, reduced fat sausages and burgers to replace fatty meat and meat product
- eating less fried food. Fat provided by chips can be reduced by using thicker cut chips; oven-chips use less fat
- eating more foods rich in iron.

POTENTIAL PROBLEMS LINKED TO POOR NUTRITION IN SCHOOLCHILDREN AND TEENAGERS

Additional resources

Healthy eating quiz from NHS Choices:
www.nhs.uk/Tools/Pages/HealthyEating.aspx?WT.srch=1
Create a weekly five-a-day friendly shopping list and meal planner in five simple steps:
www.nhs.uk/Tools/Pages/5aday.aspx?Tag=Healthy+eating
Fun healthy eating games:
www.eatwell.gov.uk/info/games

Obesity

It is estimated that about 22% of all boys and girls aged seven to 11 years in the UK can be classified as overweight, while the prevalence of obesity is around 12% in boys and 11% in girls. As with adult obesity, these levels are thought to be increasing.

There are many factors which can contribute to obesity in children, such as hormonal causes (although these are very rare), hereditary tendency, emotional factors, feeding habits in infancy, lack of physical activity, and high consumption of foods rich in fat and/or sugar. Although certain medical disorders can cause obesity, less than one per cent of all obesity is caused by physical problems.

A decrease in physical activity over recent years coupled with an abundance of energy-dense food is considered to be particularly important in explaining the increasing number of overweight children.

The causes of obesity are complex, however; basically, obesity occurs when a person eats more calories than the body burns up. In addition, if one parent is obese, there is a 50% chance that the children will also be obese. When both parents are obese, the children have an 80% chance of being obese.

 Use the NHS Choices video 'Bob is Obese' by Ian Ball to prompt discussion about lifestyle and eating:
www.nhs.uk/video/Pages/medialibrary.aspx?Tag=Healthy+eating

What are the complications of obesity?

There are many risks and complications with obesity. Physical consequences include: increased risk of heart disease, high blood pressure, diabetes, breathing problems and trouble sleeping. Child and adolescent obesity is also associated with increased risk of emotional problems. Teens with weight problems tend to have much lower self-esteem and be less popular with their peers. Depression, anxiety, and obsessive compulsive disorder can also occur

An increase in young people's levels of physical activity is not only desirable to help control body weight but also to improve health generally, including bone health and self-esteem. *See* Chapter 5 for more information on exercise.

 Additional resources

For further information on obesity, *see* the following website:
www.nationalobesityforum.org.uk

Dieting

Dramatic weight loss is not desirable while young people are still growing, and the aim should be to maintain rather than lose weight whilst height continues to increase; thus, height effectively 'catches up' with weight. A healthy, varied diet should be advocated, which might well mean the whole family must modify its eating habits. A dietitian must supervise weight reduction.

Numerous studies have reported that many teenagers, especially girls, are dissatisfied with their weight, have low self-esteem and have a distorted view of their body image. Studies have shown that up to 70% of teenage girls have attempted to lose weight—sometimes starting as young as nine years old.

In the National Diet and Nutrition Survey of Young People (2000), 16% of the girls in the 15- to 18-year-old age group were currently 'on a diet'. Such a high percentage suggests that discontent with body weight is by no means confined to overweight teenagers. It is suggested that current social pressure to conform to an 'ultra-slim' image may contribute to teenagers' dissatisfaction with their weight.

The fear of being overweight and the inappropriate eating behaviours that go along with it (e.g. fasting, skipping meals, and fad diets) are often associated with low intakes of important nutrients, such as iron and calcium. In extreme cases, more serious eating disorders such as anorexia nervosa and bulimia nervosa can develop, which are extremely damaging to health. *See* Chapter 2 for information on body image and eating disorders.

Information about diets

Dieting is not effective—Dieting changes a person's metabolism so that they are more likely to lose muscle mass than fat. Any weight lost may be put on again when the diet is stopped.

Diets stress your body—Diets that aim to drop kilos quickly actually starve the body, affecting the immune system and general well-being.

Diets can affect your emotional well-being—There is a high chance that a person will regain weight after dieting. This can lead to feelings of being a failure, self-hatred or helplessness.

Dieting makes you slow and less able to concentrate.

Vegetarianism

Vegetarianism is becoming more popular among teenagers, in particular among teenage girls. The National Diet and Nutrition Survey of Young People (2000) reported that 10% of 15- to 18-year-old girls classed themselves as vegetarian.

A vegetarian diet can be nutritionally adequate if it is carefully planned. However, problems arise if meat and fish (and eggs and dairy foods in the case of vegans) are not replaced by suitable alternatives. In a typical mixed diet, meat provides important amounts of energy, protein, vitamin B12, zinc and iron; dairy foods make a significant contribution to calcium, protein, riboflavin (vitamin B2) and vitamin B12 intake. Teenage vegetarians are particularly vulnerable to deficiency because their energy and nutrient requirements are high to support the rapid growth and development of adolescence; teenage vegans even more so because of greater restriction in food choices. Iron-deficiency anaemia is three times more common in vegetarian teenagers than non-vegetarian teenagers.

Teenagers following vegan diets are advised to take vitamin B12 supplements, since this vitamin is only found in foods of animal origin such as milk and meat. The high demand for calcium in adolescence may also necessitate calcium supplementation, especially as calcium from plant sources is relatively poorly absorbed.

Sport

Exercise is considered essential for healthy growth and development and, as discussed above, the majority of children and teenagers in the UK should increase their levels of activity. However, some young people are involved in competitive sport and accompanying intensive training schedules. This sort of exercise adds additional energy and nutritional costs to the already high requirements of adolescence and can therefore increase the risk of dietary inadequacy.

Low intakes of energy and nutrients, including calcium and iron, are particularly common in female athletes who are restricting their food intake in order to maintain a low body weight (e.g. gymnasts, long distance runners and lightweight rowers). Teenagers who participate in sports where the typical body weight is heavier are more likely to have adequate diets. Low calcium intakes, coupled with menstrual abnormalities, can have a deleterious effect on bone health.

Body mass index

 Get your group members to measure their BMI (each young person should do this individually, as weight can be a sensitive issue). Use the web link in the following box to calculate BMI. Use a handout to inform the young people where their weight falls within the BMI index.

Using body mass index (BMI) for a healthy weight

BMI is a measure that allows you to check if your weight is healthy for your height. It allows for natural variations in body shape, giving a healthy weight range for a particular height.

Use the chart or the following website to calculate your BMI: www.nhs.uk/Tools/Pages/Healthyweightcalculator.aspx?Tag= (or the chart on the following page)

BMI 18.5–24.9

The ideal weight-for-height range. A BMI below 18.5 is a health risk and too low for optimal health.

BMI 25.0–29.9

Weight just above the ideal range. Check your diet and make small changes to prevent more weight gain and to help lose the extra weight.

BMI 30.0–34.9

Dietary changes required immediately. Higher risk of developing ill health due to weight; 10 times more likely to get diabetes; increasing risk of arthritis, heart disease and some cancers. This means a shorter life expectancy, and weight-related health concerns reducing quality of life.

BMI 35.0+

Weight seriously affecting health. Raised risk of heart disease, stroke and premature death. In addition to making lifestyle changes, weight should be discussed with a GP or nurse, as the additional support of a health professional may be required.

BODY MASS INDEX CHART

Height in feet / inches

Weight	4'10	5'0	5'2	5'4	5'6	5'8	5'10	6'0	6'2	6'4
7st 0	20.6	19.2	18.0	16.9	15.9	15.0	14.1	13.3	12.6	—
7st 7	22.0	20.6	19.3	18.1	17.0	16.0	15.1	14.3	13.5	12.8
8st 0	23.5	22.0	20.6	19.3	18.1	17.1	16.1	15.2	14.4	13.7
8st 7	25.0	23.3	21.8	20.5	19.3	18.2	17.1	16.2	15.3	14.5
9st 0	26.4	24.7	23.1	21.7	20.4	19.2	18.1	17.2	16.2	15.4
9st 7	27.9	26.1	24.4	22.9	21.5	20.3	19.2	18.1	17.1	16.2
10st 0	29.4	27.4	25.7	24.1	22.7	21.4	20.2	19.1	18.0	17.1
10st 7	30.8	28.8	27.0	25.3	23.8	22.4	21.2	20.0	18.9	18.0
11st 0	32.3	30.2	28.3	26.5	24.9	23.5	22.2	21.0	19.8	18.8
11st 7	33.8	31.6	29.6	27.7	26.1	24.6	23.2	21.9	20.7	19.7
12st 0	35.2	32.9	30.8	28.9	27.2	25.6	24.2	22.9	21.6	20.5
12st 7	36.7	34.3	32.1	30.1	28.3	26.7	25.2	23.8	22.5	21.4
13st 0	38.2	35.7	33.4	31.4	29.5	27.8	26.2	24.8	23.5	22.2
13st 7	39.6	37.0	34.7	32.6	30.6	28.8	27.2	25.7	24.4	23.1
14st 0	41.1	38.4	36.0	33.8	31.7	29.9	28.2	26.7	25.3	23.9
14st 7	42.6	39.8	37.3	35.0	32.9	31.0	29.2	27.6	26.2	24.8
15st 0	44.0	41.2	38.5	36.2	34.0	32.0	30.2	28.6	27.1	25.7
15st 7	45.5	42.5	39.8	37.4	35.2	33.1	31.2	29.5	28.0	26.5
16st 0	47.0	43.9	41.1	38.6	36.3	34.2	32.3	30.5	28.9	27.4
16st 7	48.5	45.3	42.4	39.8	37.4	35.2	33.3	31.4	29.8	28.2
17st 0	49.9	46.6	43.7	41.0	38.6	36.3	34.3	32.4	30.7	29.1
17st 7	51.4	48.0	45.0	42.2	39.7	37.4	35.3	33.3	31.6	29.9
18st 0	52.9	49.4	46.3	43.4	40.8	38.5	36.3	34.3	32.5	30.8
18st 7	54.3	50.8	47.5	44.6	42.0	39.5	37.3	35.3	33.4	31.6
19st 0	55.8	52.1	48.8	45.8	43.1	40.6	38.3	36.2	34.3	32.5
19st 7	57.3	53.5	50.1	47.0	44.2	41.7	39.3	37.2	35.2	33.3
20st 0	58.7	54.9	51.4	48.2	45.4	42.7	40.3	38.1	36.1	34.2
Stones/Lbs	4'10	5'0	5'2	5'4	5'6	5'8	5'10	6'0	6'2	6'4

Make smoothies

Use bananas to add sweetness, not sugar nor honey. Get the group to be creative with their fruit (or even vegetable) combinations.

Healthy snack recipes:

Chocolate balls

75 g butter
150 mL blended dates
1 tbsp vanilla essence
2–3 tbsp cocoa
600 mL oats

Pour hot water over pitted dates. Blend. Add other ingredients. Roll into small balls; coat in cocoa powder. Chill in fridge.

Banana cookies

Take three bananas (mashed).
Add oats until the mixture is stiff.
Add raisins, nuts, cinnamon, and ginger to taste.
Bake in the oven 10–15 minutes at 200 C/400 F/GM6.

Additional resources

Step-by-step cooking guide:
www.bbc.co.uk/food/get_cooking

Play interactive healthy eating games on the following website:
www.nourishinteractive.com

Make a balanced plate and other activities:
www.foodafactoflife.org.uk

CHAPTER 5

Exercise

The area of exercise and young people is inextricably linked to healthy eating. Basically, to maintain a healthy weight, all calories taken in need to be used up through body function or exercise, otherwise the individual will gain weight. Naturally there are other benefits too, e.g. a healthy heart, a good level of fitness and the positive mood effects of exercise.

Many factors conspire to make adolescence a time where regular exercise is shelved: working towards exams, worry over body image and not wanting others to see you in gym clothes, as well as the increasing use of the internet, game consoles and general fears over safety if out and about.

Who is at risk?

Research shows that priority groups for obesity are:
- girls aged 12–18 years
- young people of low socio-economic status
- young people 16–18 years
- those from black and ethnic minority groups
- those with physical and mental disabilities
- those with clinical conditions such as depression or diabetes.

Print the following sheet to prompt a group discussion regarding what contributes to teenagers exercising less:

'I think that the physical education in school is generally quite poor. Year seven, eight and nine pupils are quite enthusiastic. However, in year ten 10 and 11, with the added pressure of GCSEs, pupils can't be bothered to do this compulsory activity.'

'I think that generally we are getting slack at keeping fit and I would blame it on the new game consoles, TV channels and computers becoming available to us. We are getting addicted to them and instead of spending time in the local park playing football, riding our bikes, or skateboarding, we're doing it on our Play Station, Dreamcast, or Nintendo instead.'

'Sometimes this is due to using time more effectively; sometimes because young people feel embarrassed due to their size or physical fitness or don't feel that the activities hold anything they would like to do.'

Schools and colleges need to have a wider range of activities for young people to try and entice them into doing more physical activities. These things could include regular visits to the leisure centre to have the option of swimming, badminton, tennis, etc.

Source: *Headliners* at www.**headliners**.org

JOINED UP ACTION

The previous government identified the health needs of teenagers as a priority area in the *Choosing Health White Paper*. The need to support children and young people, as well as their parents, carers and families in the development of a 'healthy framework for life' was recognised. A broad programme of initiatives was instigated to provide this support. Fundamental to this programme was the drive to ensure that health services are equipped and coordinated to meet children and young people's needs. *Choosing Health* built on the requirements set out in the Children, Young People and Maternity Services National Service Framework, which aim to make healthcare provision accessible and welcoming to young people.

In addition, one of the Every Child Matters statutes is to facilitate 'staying healthy', which would include laying foundations for future health, one aspect of which would be facilitating exercise opportunities for young people.

Schools are taking an active part in this process; the majority subscribe to the National Healthy Schools Programme, which takes a holistic approach to young people's health.

The National Healthy Schools Programme is an exciting long-term initiative that is making a significant difference to the health and achievement of children and young people. The programme supports the links between health, behaviour and achievement; it is about creating healthy and happy children and young people who do better in learning and in life.

The impact of the programme is based on a whole-school approach to physical and emotional well-being focused on four core themes:

- personal, social and health education
- healthy eating
- physical activity
- emotional health and well-being.

Source: National Healthy School Standard (DfEE 1999)

Why bother exercising?

- Physical inactivity is an independent risk factor for coronary heart disease—in other words, if you don't exercise you dramatically increase your risk of dying from a heart attack.
- Exercise means a healthier heart because it reduces several cardiovascular risks, including high blood pressure.
- Being physically active can bolster good mental health and help you to manage stress, anxiety and even depression.
- Regular exercise can help you achieve and maintain an ideal weight, which can be important in managing many health conditions, or may just make you feel happier about your appearance.
- All exercise helps strengthen bones and muscles to some degree, but weight-bearing exercise, such as running, is especially good in promoting bone density and protecting against osteoporosis, which affects men as well as women.
- Different exercises help with all sorts of health niggles, such as digestion, poor posture and sleeplessness. Physical activity can be beneficial for a range of medical conditions, from diabetes to lower back pain.

How much exercise do I need?

- *It is recommended that children and young people get one hour of physical activity a day.*
- This activity should be of at least moderate intensity—in other words, you should work up a bit of a sweat and get slightly out of breath. But if you can manage something a bit more strenuous, then that's even better.
- At least twice a week you should include activities to improve bone health, muscle strength and flexibility. Activities that are 'weight bearing' (in other words, where you are on your feet, rather than in water or on a bike) help build strong bones.

 Print the following quiz for your group to do individually—get them thinking about simple areas where they might be able to improve their diet and exercise routines.

HOW HEALTHY ARE YOU?

Fill out the questionnaire to find out how healthy you are.

Food and drink

		A	B	C	D
1	How many servings of fruits and vegetables do you eat each day?	0	1–2	3–4	5 plus
2	Do you eat breakfast?	Never	Occasionally	Most days	Daily
3	Do you miss out on other meals?	Daily	Most days	Occasionally	Never
4	How many glasses of water do you drink a day?	0–1	2–3	4–5	6–8
5	How many glasses of fizzy drinks (e.g. Coke) do you drink per day?	3 or more	2	1	0
6	How often do you eat sweets/cakes?	Daily	Most days	Occasionally	Never
7	How often do you eat crisps or other savoury snack foods?	Daily	Most days	Occasionally	Never
8	How often do you eat takeaway foods (chips, burgers, kebabs, etc.)?	Daily	Most days	Occasionally	Never
9	How many times do you eat/drink milk, cheese or yoghurt?	Never	1–2 times a week	Once a day	2–3 times a day

Activity

	A	B	C	D
1 How many times do you walk to work/school?	Never	Few times each month	Few times each week	Daily
2 How do you get to work/school?	Car	Bus or train	Walk or cycle	
3 How many hours of television do you watch each day?	4 or more	3	2	0–1
4 How many hours do you spend on your computer each day?	4 or more	3	2	0–1
5 How often do you exercise?	Never	Few times each month	Few times each week	Daily
6 If at school, how often do you participate in PE?	Never	Few times each month	Few times each week	Daily
7 Do you go to any after-school/leisure centre or do other activities such as dance, swimming or judo?	Never	Few times each month	Few times each week	Daily

Thank you for doing the quiz. Now—how healthy are you?

Mostly A's   Ooh, at the moment your food intake and activity levels could be a bit healthier. Take a look at your answers. What could you change? Walk part of the way to school/work; increase the amount of fruit you eat; cut down on fats and sugars; drink water instead of fizzy drinks?

Mostly B's   You've made some good choices, but there is still room for improvement. Take a look at your answers. How could you have more C's and D's? Think about it. Are you getting a balance of activity levels?

Mostly C's   That's really quite good, but there are always ways to be even healthier! What could you change?

Mostly D's   Well done! Your diet and activity levels look very good. Keep up the good work!

With thanks to Samina Tarafder, Public Health, City and Hackney Community Health Services.

ACTIVITIES TO ASSESS FITNESS LEVELS

Resting heart rate

As fitness improves, resting heart rate (RHR) will decrease. Measure your heart rate while still in bed, first thing in the morning. It is easiest to just count how many times your heart beats in one minute (60 seconds). This is typically between 50 to 100 beats in one minute (bpm). Athletes have lower resting heart rates, while sedentary people have higher resting heart rates.

Measuring body fat distribution

The waist-to-hip ratio (WHR) tells you whether you have a healthier body fat distribution. Research is finding that abdominal fat is an indicator of higher risk for diseases such as chronic heart failure. Measure your waist and then your hips, and divide the waist measurement by the hip measurement (units don't matter; you can use either inches or centimetres). In women, the ratio should be 0.8 or less, and in men it should be 1.0 or less.

Measuring total body fat

You can measure total body fat with several methods, including a body fat scale, a skinfold test with calipers, an immersion test, or by taking several measurements and calculating. This body fat measurement is a better indicator than simply weighing yourself. This is best done in the context of a consultation with a dietician.

SO WHAT SORT OF EXERCISE CAN I DO?

Getting fit isn't all about gyms—some forms of exercise won't cost you a penny, and most types can easily be slotted into a busy lifestyle without having to find a few extra hours in your day.

Walking

Most of us walk at some point each day, but we do it far less than we used to—yet walking is the simplest and cheapest of all exercises; making it a regular activity and focusing on the intensity or distance covered can greatly increase fitness.

Walking improves the condition of your heart and lungs (cardiovascular fitness) and works the muscles of the lower body. It's a weight-bearing activity, so it may improve bone density, yet it's also low impact, putting less stress on the joints than some other forms of exercise.

Running/jogging

Running might just be the ultimate way to get fit: it's cheap and can be done anywhere, at any time and, most importantly, it is very effective. There's really no difference between running and jogging, although jogging is often used to describe running at a slow pace. Whatever you call it, all you need is a good pair of running shoes and a little enthusiasm.

As a high-impact activity, running may maintain or increase bone density, helping to offset osteoporosis. But it can also put more stress on your joints than lower impact activities such as walking and cycling, especially if you're overweight.

How to run …

As with all exercise, you must warm up first. Start by walking at a brisk pace, then gradually break into a slow jog. Run at a pace at which you can still hold a conversation, but which definitely feels harder than walking. If you're getting too breathless to talk, slow down or walk for a while until you're breathing more easily.

To begin with, aim to run/walk in this way for 10 minutes in total. Do this every second or third day, gradually reducing the walking time and increasing the running until you can run for the full 10 minutes.

At the end of each session, cool down by finishing with a slow jog or brisk walk until your heart rate and breathing have returned to more normal levels. Stretch while your muscles are still warm.

Next, start to increase the total duration of your run by a minute or two every third session, until you can manage 30 minutes three times a week. Even if you're feeling good, don't be tempted to increase your running time by more than 10% each week.

Many people are put off running because they find it boring. For this reason, it is important to get a bit of variety in your running. There are many different sorts of running: road running, cross-country running, fell running (running in the hills), or you could run at your local athletics track, or even on a treadmill at the gym (though running on a moving treadmill uses less energy). Other tips to stay motivated include:

- have a clear aim, such as competing in a local fun run or being able to run non-stop for an hour
- be realistic—don't commit to running a marathon in three months if you've never run before
- think of yourself as a runner and make running a habit, just like cleaning your teeth—think in terms of 'when I go for my run' rather than 'if I go for a run'
- keep a diary—record your progress, the time of day, the weather, how you felt, where you went and so on.

Swimming

Swimming is another popular way to start getting fit because most towns have a relatively inexpensive pool, and you need even less of a kit than you do for running. Most pools also offer lessons if you're a non-swimmer, or if you haven't swum for years and want to improve your technique.

Swimming is a great way to tone up and trim down, because to swim you need to move your body against the resistance of the water. Just swimming a few lengths involves most of the major muscle groups, giving your body a good workout. And if you crank up the pace, you'll get a brilliant aerobic workout too.

Swimming is also an effective form of fat-burning exercise: because you can swim at your own pace: you keep swimming for long periods and maintaining your staying power is a vital goal in fat-burning exercise.

The other big advantage is that water supports your weight and takes the stress off your joints, so you can put your body through a good workout without your knees, hips or spine paying the price.

Research shows that exercising in waist-deep water reduces the pressure on joints by 50%, while exercising in chest-deep water reduces it by as much as 75%. This can also make it a great exercise if you're recovering from an injury and you can't run or play your normal sport.

Cycling

Some of the main benefits of cycling are:

- **a healthy heart**—A major study of more than 10 000 people found those who cycle at least 20 miles a week are half as likely to have heart problems as those who don't cycle at all
- **weight control**—Some research suggests we should be burning up at least 2 000 calories a week through exercise (actually far more than used by the recommended 30 minutes of moderately intensive exercise five times a week). Cycling burns about 300 calories an hour, so if you do it twice a day, the numbers soon add up
- **it can be part of your routine**—If you're worried about making time for exercise, why not see whether it's feasible to cycle to and from school/college, which would incorporate excellent exercise into your normal daily routine
- Because the bicycle supports your body, cycling isn't necessarily a weight-bearing exercise. This means it's good for people with certain bone and joint problems because it puts very little pressure on these body parts—but it also makes it less effective for protecting against osteoporosis.

Team sports

Getting fit isn't just something you have to do by yourself. Playing team sports like football, hockey or netball is great exercise, and is often more enjoyable because you're with a group of friends.

Your school or college may run sessions in the evening, or you might want to get involved with a local team. You can find details of local clubs on the internet, in the phone book or at your nearest leisure centre. Your local authority can also give you information on sporting activities in your area.

Activities you can introduce in your group:

Using a pedometer
Give your group pedometers and instructions in how to use them—the aim is to make 10 000 steps a day.

Remember: *Taking 10 000 steps burns 500 calories*

Research has shown that this step-counting gadget, worn at the waist, is a surprisingly effective encouragement for people to be more active. A pedometer gives the user the ability to measure how much he or she has done and a goal to aspire to. Walking the recommended 10 000 steps in a day will burn 500 calories, and doing that five days a week will burn 3 500 calories—enough to lose 500 g (1 lb) of body fat.

Skipping
Skipping can be used for several reasons in respect to your fitness. For example, it can help with endurance training or to develop your speed in short bursts. It is also an excellent exercise to help you train your coordination and to develop a sense of rhythm.

Skipping is excellent because it is a cheap, medium impact exercise and extremely effective for improving your cardiovascular fitness.

Skipping will help improve cardio-respiratory (heart and lung) fitness, flexibility and co-ordination, and can help reduce the risk of heart disease and lower blood pressure and cholesterol levels. It's also an excellent way for you to lose weight or tone up.

The basics of skipping

- Always make sure that you skip whilst wearing properly fitting trainers, as this will help to support your feet, ankles and also your knees.
- Ensure that you keep your elbows tucked in and do not lean forward.
- Try to skip quickly, but keep your movements to a minimum. You want to keep the rope tight.
- Alternate jumping from one foot to the other whilst skipping the rope. Do not jump the rope with both feet together. Try to be light on your feet and land softly with each foot.
- At first it is a good idea to try to skip for at least a minute and then take a three-minute rest.
- It's also a good idea to skip with music playing, which will help you to keep going.

 Have a noticeboard in your organisation that has details of local sports/fitness classes and swim timetables.

 Invite a trainer to your organisation to do a taster session in aerobics, kick boxing or another sport so your young people can get a feel for an activity without having to go alone and sign up.

 Set up a regular class on your premises and encourage young people to go; in fact, attend yourself!

Play games!

Incorporating games into your youth club or group schedule can be a good way to include exercise in your programme. Team games are best, where there is not a focus on individual performance. For example:

 Relay races

Teens are divided into groups of equal numbers. Each team member takes a turn running a leg of the race until one team crosses the finish line.

Tug of war

Teens are divided into two groups, attempting to create groups of approximately the same strength. A line is marked on the ground, with teams placed on opposite sides of the line. All team members grasp a long length of rope and attempt to pull the members of the opposing team across the dividing line.

Silly string tag

This game is so simple and easy, yet kids love it because it adds just a little something different. You play tag (or even freeze tag) just like you normally would, except that whoever is 'it' is armed with a can of silly string (the spray string you get in party shops). You must be hit with the silly string to be 'it'. Once someone else is 'it', the can is passed to that person and so on. Be sure to have some extra cans on hand, because once they start playing, they won't want to stop!

Additional resources

Watch the NHS Choices video 'Activity Sinners and Saints': http://tinyurl.com/yd8g56b

GIRLS AND EXERCISE

Most girls reduce their rate of physical activity once they reach the teen years. This explains why the incidence of young women being overweight and obese tends to double during adolescence, even though eating habits may remain the same. An overweight teenager is likely to become an overweight adult who risks obesity—related conditions such as cardiovascular disease and diabetes. A teenage girl's level of physical activity has a direct influence on her weight.

COMMON BARRIERS

Some of the reasons why teenage girls might avoid exercise and sport include:
- physically inactive parents who model sedentary behaviours
- lack of energy due to poor physical fitness
- the myth that you can't be 'feminine' and play sport
- peer pressure, such as having friends who don't exercise or play sport
- lack of basic skills (such as throwing and catching a ball)
- fear of feeling incompetent on the field

- fear of looking silly in front of other people, especially peers
- fear of being teased or mocked by other players for being unskilled
- previous bad experiences during physical education class (such as teasing from peers)
- embarrassment about wearing sporting uniforms (such as swimming costumes or short skirts).

HOW TO ENCOURAGE YOUNG WOMEN TO EXERCISE

- **Talk about it**—Ask what bothers her about exercise. Understanding the reasons why she avoids exercise is important because it can help you discuss possible solutions. For example, if she is shy of revealing her body, don't suggest that she try swimming. Instead, pick an activity that can be performed wearing tracksuit trousers and a T-shirt.
- **Be a role model**—Exercise yourself, if you don't already. Show her how keeping fit is fun and rewarding. Girls who have physically active role models are much more likely to exercise.
- **Watch women's sports**—Attend sporting matches together or watch them on television. Show her that sport isn't a male domain.
- **Teach the skills**—Explain the rules and jargon of different sports. Help her practice physical skills such as throwing and catching a ball.
- **Have fun**—Inactive girls tend to think of exercise as boring hard work. Try to show her that exercise can be fun. Experiment with pleasurable activities such as dance or rollerblading.
- **Keep it simple**—Emphasise that physical activity is not just sport or going to the gym and that it doesn't need to be a structured activity. It can be integrated into daily routines through walking, using stairs, walking the dog, cycling and so on.

HOW CAN YOU GET THE MOST OUT OF EXERCISE?

Exercise helps the body the most when a person:
- eats healthy foods, following the balance of good health 'plate' (*see* Chapter 4)
- gets enough sleep so the body has time to rest and recover between workouts
- avoids anabolic steroids, which are powerful chemicals that can cause liver problems and increase the risk for high blood pressure, heart attack and stroke.

Steroids

Anabolic steroids are synthetic compounds that mimic the action of the male sex hormone testosterone. The drugs have some medical uses, but some athletes and sports enthusiasts do abuse them because they want to increase muscle mass and improve performance. Some teens use steroids because of concern about body image.

In adolescents, anabolic steroid abuse can halt bone growth and has been associated with damage to the heart, kidneys and liver. In males, steroid abuse can lead to impotence, shrunken testicles and breast enlargement. In females, the drugs' effects include menstrual irregularities, growth of body hair and loss of scalp hair, a deepened voice and reduction in breast size. Some of these biological effects are irreversible. Use of anabolic steroids also has been linked to increased and unpredictable levels of aggression in human and animal studies.

Additional resources

For more detail on steroids, visit the 'Talk to Frank' website: www.talktofrank.com

---

Overexercising

How do you know if your fitness routine is out of control? The main difference between a healthy exercise habit and a dependence on exercise is how the exercise fits into your life. If you put workouts ahead of friends, homework and other responsibilities, you may be developing a dependence on exercise.

If you are concerned about your own exercise habits or a friend's, ask yourself the following questions. Do you:
• force yourself to exercise, even if you don't feel well?
• prefer to exercise rather than being with friends?
• become very upset if you miss a workout?
• base the amount you exercise on how much you eat?
• have trouble sitting still because you think you're not burning calories?
• worry that you'll gain weight if you skip exercising for a day?

Girls and boys who exercise compulsively may have a distorted body image and low self-esteem. They may see themselves as overweight or out of shape even when they are actually a healthy weight.

If you feel you may be overexercising:
• work on changing your daily self-talk. When you look in the mirror, make sure you find at least one good thing to say about yourself. Be more aware of your positive attributes
• when you exercise, focus on the positive, mood-boosting qualities
• give yourself a break. Listen to your body and give yourself a day of rest after a hard workout
• control your weight by exercising and eating moderate portions of healthy foods. Don't try to change your body into an unrealistically lean shape. Talk with your doctor, dietitian, coach, trainer or other adult about what a healthy body weight is for you and how to develop healthy eating and exercise habits.

CHAPTER 6

What's your poison?

Smoking, alcohol and drugs

There is general consensus that abuse of drugs and alcohol can result in poor health and social outcomes. In addition to the much-publicised possible mental health effects, being under the influence of drugs or alcohol can impair decision making and lead young people to do things that they may regret, e.g. having sex, having unprotected sex, getting involved in petty crime, etc.

The debate over the legalities of various substances and their use is fraught and regularly makes the headlines. Only recently the labour government reclassified cannabis back to a class B drug, after only a few years of classification as a class C drug. Messages are mixed and are understandably confusing; you cannot buy cigarettes or alcohol until aged 18, although you can drink alcohol in certain circumstances under that age. Although cannabis is illegal, punishments vary according to whether it is for personal use or for sale; medication such as Valium can be prescribed for certain conditions but cannot be used 'recreationally'; magic mushrooms are legal if prepared one way and illegal in another …

Even with all this varying and changing legislation, naturally the overarching aim is to reduce harm to individuals. The aim of work with young people should be to raise their awareness of these issues and the facts around substance use and misuse so they can make informed decisions for themselves.

Professionals working with young people should have a basic knowledge of the different drugs, their effects and the possible consequences of their use both physically and legally.

This chapter will outline the government strategies that inform our practice, statistics regarding young people and drug use, and how information we give aligns with the school curriculum. Photocopiable information sheets will outline what the different drugs are, the drugs' effects, and the legal stance on each drug, with suggested activities to explore young people's knowledge of and attitudes towards drugs.

Some facts ...

- The prevalence of drug use is higher among boys than girls.
- 15% of boys aged 11 to 15 years had used drugs in the last year compared with 13% of girls, and 31% of males aged 16 to 19 years used drugs in the last year compared with 24% of females in the same age group.
- Cannabis is the most widely used drug among 11 to 19 year olds.
  - of those aged 11 to 15 years in England, 12% were using cannabis. In England and Wales, 25% of those aged 16 to 19 years were using cannabis. The prevalence of using cannabis and class A drugs increased with age.
- The use of amphetamines, LSD and poppers has decreased among 16 to 19 year olds.
- Girls are more likely to smoke than boys among those aged 11 to 15 years.
- 12% of girls aged 11 to 15 years in England are regular smokers compared with 9% of boys.
  - However, in this age group, consumption of cigarettes among regular smokers was higher for boys than girls, with boys smoking an average of 50 cigarettes in a week compared with 44 for girls.
- In England, the prevalence of drinking alcohol in the last week for all young people aged 11 to 15 years increased slightly from 21% in 1990 to 24% in 2000.
- Boys were more likely than girls to have consumed alcohol in the last week: 25% of boys consumed, compared with 23% of girls. Boys aged 11 to 15 years were likely to consume more units of alcohol than girls in the same age group. The average consumption for boys was 11.6 units compared with 9.1 units for girls. Beer, lager and cider were the most popular types of alcohol in both boys and girls.

Source: www.statistics.gov.uk/cci/nugget.asp?id=719 (2000)

What does the government say?

Reducing drug use by young people, particularly the most vulnerable, is central to the government's updated National Drug Strategy.

Additional resources

The Home Office's Drugs and Alcohol page:
http://drugs.homeoffice.gov.uk/young-people

Drug Action Teams (DATs)

The government has instigated drug action teams. A central part of the National Drug Strategy, these are local strategic partnerships responsible for delivering the National Drugs Strategy at a local level.

DATs take strategic decisions on expenditure and service delivery within the four aims of the National Drugs Strategy. Those four aims are:

1 **Treatment**—Reducing drug use and drug-related offending through treatment and support; reducing drug-related death through harm minimisation
2 **Young people**—Preventing today's young people from becoming tomorrow's problematic drug users
3 **Communities**—Reducing drug-related crime and its impact on communities
4 **Supply**—Reducing the supply of illegal drugs.

DATs ensure that the work of local agencies tackling drug misuse is brought together effectively, and that cross-agency projects are coordinated successfully.

DATs bring together representatives of key local agencies. These are likely to include:

- health
- social services
- the police
- probation
- the prison service
- education
- connexions
- youth offending teams
- housing
- voluntary sector agencies.

DATs are formally accountable to the Home Secretary. They are supported by Home Office teams in the nine regional government offices, and centrally by the Drugs Strategy Directorate, which is based within the Home Office.

What's in the curriculum?

At secondary school, drug education will normally be part of a combined Personal Social Health and Economic (PSHE) education programme. It will build on the provision at the primary level to complete drug education in school. For professionals working with young people, it gives guidance on what knowledge is recommended at which age. As with sexual health education, when tackling drug awareness in a group it is recommended that you follow the PSHE guidance and inform parents that this subject is going to be covered (it might be worth running a session for parents and/or providing information for them, as this is an area that parents often do not feel confident tackling with their children).

By the end of S2 (years 3–6; ages 7–10), pupils will learn:
- about the range of drugs and the effects and consequences (medical and legal) of drug misuse, including drugs in sport
- that drugs are much more likely to cause health problems when using more than one at the same time
- that the effects of drugs are often unpredictable, or develop gradually without the user realising it
- the school policy regarding drug misuse by pupils
- the impact that healthy and unhealthy choices can have on their lives
- decision-making skills to allow them to make positive choices about their health
- that life involves taking risks and some are to be avoided as they can harm health
- about the law relating to drugs, tobacco and alcohol
- how to access local health support services.

By the end of S4 (years 10 and 11; ages 14–16), pupils will also learn:
- symptoms of drug misuse
- the social cost of drug misuse
- that drugs have an effect on behaviour and ability to make decisions
- that infection can be spread by drug apparatus, including used needles
- skills of self-control, self-confidence and assertiveness to allow them to be in control of their own lives
- the value of fitness for health in adult life, and that drugs would threaten this
- that drugs, alcohol and tobacco can affect the development of the human embryo.

Core drug education should be completed by the end of S4, since this is the time when pupils start reaching the end of their school years. By this time pupils should be equipped with the knowledge and skills they need to avoid misusing drugs.

SMOKING

Smoking statistics

- Every year around 200,000 children and young people start smoking regularly, approximately 550 a day.
- Girls are more likely than boys to have ever smoked and to be regular smokers.
- Children who live with parents or siblings who smoke are around 90% more likely to become smokers themselves than children of non smoking households.
- There is a strong association between smoking and other substance use ie drugs and alcohol.

Young smokers are at serious risk of poor respiratory health in both the short and long term: coughs, increased phlegm, wheeziness, shortness of breath, impairment of lung growth, chronic obstructive pulmonary disease in later life, lung cancer and heart disease.

Source: *Ash: essential information on young people and smoking*. Available at: www.ash.org.uk (January 2011).

Smoking prevention for young people

There is very little evidence on what works to reduce smoking and smoking uptake among young people. The emphasis at present is on working with adults, which ultimately protects children from exposure to tobacco smoke and promotes quitting by adults (and parents in particular)—this in turn reduces the likelihood of children taking up smoking.

Having said that, there is some evidence that peer interventions can have an effect in reducing smoking; non-smoking policies generally reinforce non-smoking as the norm in society. Thus, school-based prevention programmes that draw on multiple strategies can be effective in reducing tobacco use.

Other national interventions that have been effective in reducing smoking prevalence are reducing the sale of tobacco to those under age 16 (and more recently under age 18), mass media anti-smoking campaigns, increasing the number of smoke-free public places and increasing the price of cigarettes.

For professionals working with young people, it can be helpful to stress how smoking can negatively affect other areas in their lives that are important to them, e.g. attracting a partner and fitness and performance.

Have a discussion with your group about the physical effects of smoking on the body. Gory pictures from the Internet, whilst not proven to actually motivate people to stop smoking, are certainly a conversation starter. The following hand-outs can be given out, or be displayed on a youth noticeboard where the messages are constantly reinforced rather than put in the bin or lost!

What are the effects of smoking on your body?

- Over 120,000 people die each year from smoking-related diseases. That is 330 people each day—**the equivalent of a jumbo jet crashing every day of the year!**
- Over half of today's young smokers will eventually be killed by their habit.
- One in five UK deaths is caused by smoking.
- Smoking causes 10 times more deaths than road accidents (3 000), infectious diseases (2 000), liver cirrhosis (3 000) and suicide (4 000) combined together.
- The risk of a having a heart attack is greater in smokers than non-smokers.
- Thirty per cent of all cancer deaths are attributed to smoking. Cancers linked to smoking include: lung cancer; cervical cancer; cancers of the mouth, lip and throat; cancer of the pancreas, bladder cancer, stomach cancer, cancer of the kidney and liver cancer.
- Smoking causes approximately 82% of all deaths from lung cancer, 83% of all deaths from bronchitis and emphysema and about 25% of all deaths from heart disease.
- Smoking causes about 90% of peripheral vascular disease, which leads to about 2 000 leg amputations each year.

Smoking and fitness

Smoking reduces fitness and sporting performance. If you smoke or use tobacco products, you are not going to be able to run as fast or as far as your smoke-free teammates.

Tobacco slows down your lung growth and reduces lung function, which can leave you gulping for air when you need it most.

Young smokers suffer from shortness of breath almost three times as often as those who do not smoke.

A smoker's heart has to work much harder than that of a non-smoker. So in competition, your body wastes a lot more energy just trying to keep up with non-smokers.

What is happening to your body when you smoke?

- High levels of carbon monoxide from smoking reduce the amount of oxygen absorbed into the blood from the lungs. You then have to breathe faster and deeper to get a good amount of oxygen to your blood. This makes you breathless and tired much sooner than a non-smoker.
- Carbon monoxide in the blood reduces the amount of oxygen that is released from the blood into the muscles. This means you get more tired more quickly and may not be able to achieve as much as a non-smoker.
- Blood levels of carbon monoxide from smoking can also produce distortions of time perception, psychomotor and visual impairment and negative effects on cognitive skill. It can make you less physically able and less intelligent.
- Smoke inhalation has an immediate effect on breathing, reducing airway elasticity, increasing your airway resistance and therefore reducing the amount of oxygen absorbed into the blood.
- Smoking causes chronic (long-term) swelling of mucous membranes, which also leads to increased airway resistance and reduced oxygen to the blood.
- The tar in cigarettes coats the lungs, reducing the elasticity of the air sacs and resulting in the absorption of less oxygen into the blood stream.
- Tar also affects the cleansing mechanism of the lungs, allowing pollutants to remain in the bronchial tubes and lungs. Increased phlegm and coughing, and damage to the cilia (the hair-like projections which 'sweep' pollutants out of the airways) are the result.

National 'No Smoking Day happens every year in March. Mark this occasion. Your local health care provider will only be too happy to provide you with materials to bring the event to life, and will most likely be running a campaign that could include a 'quit smoking' team having an event at your venue. If you are unsure who to contact, call the national quitline, and they will point you in the right direction.

The National Quitline: 0800 022 4332

If you have a young person (or indeed someone of any age) who would like to stop smoking, offer plenty of encouragement and direct the person to his GP/Practice Nurse/Pharmacy, who will be able to take him through the quitting process as well as provide nicotine replacement therapy (NRT). NRT is not a magic cure; however, attempting to give up with a form of NRT makes the process twice as likely to be successful. If it is an area about which you feel particularly enthusiastic, many PCTs offer training in smoking cessation for non-health professionals, enabling them to provide appropriate counselling as well as the ability to provide NRT. Again, call the number above to link into this training.

How to quit smoking

1 Pick a date to stop.
2 List your reasons for stopping.
3 Ask a friend to quit, and support each other.
4 Keep busy—find something else to do.
5 Try some exercise—you will feel fitter. This can also help prevent any weight gain.
6 Drink more water; it helps with cravings.
7 Be positive and think: 'I can do it!'
8 Get some professional support; you are twice a likely to stop if using a nicotine replacement product (e.g. patches or gum).

The benefits of stopping smoking

The benefits of being smoke-free include the following:
- healthy lungs, heart and blood
- it's easier to breathe
- fitness—you won't be exhausted when exercising
- fresh breath—you'll be more 'kissable'
- clean hair and clothes
- better sense of taste and smell
- nicotine-free teeth and fingers
- fresh looks—no wrinkles!
- feeling healthy and positive
- more money—extra cash to buy your favourite things, such as CDs, computer games, make-up, sporting goods, mobile phone top-up cards and magazines.

Draw a rough diagram of a young person on flip-chart paper.
Get the group to brainstorm why a young person might smoke.
  For example, answers might include: it's cool, it gives a better image, smoking makes you popular or attractive, it reduces stress, it controls weight, TV/movie/music personalities do it, etc.

Add in other issues they may not have included, such as low self-esteem, poor self-image and lack of confidence in one's self to say 'no' when someone wants them to try smoking.

Brainstorm the inner-body health problems from smoking, e.g. shortness of breath, coughing, nausea and dizziness. Shade in areas of the body that are affected by smoking.

Look at those areas that could be affected later in life if 'The Smoker' continues to smoke (e.g. cancer of the lungs and other areas of the body, heart disease, damage to the respiratory system, added strain on the heart, narrowing of blood vessels and stroke).

Brainstorm outer-body health problems from smoking (e.g. bad breath, discoloured teeth, stinky hair and clothes, cracking lips and mouth sores. The Smoker will also have problems in sports—he/she will run slower and have weak muscles. Shade in these areas of the body that are affected by smoking.

Finally, discuss how the smoker affects others when he/she smokes, e.g. secondhand smoke, illness, death, fires.

Invite a 'stop smoking' advisor from your local primary care trust to come and speak with your group. This can be useful, as it links young people into support organisations. The advisor usually has access to good visual aids as well, which bring the reality of the effects of smoking to life.

The National Quitline (0800 022 4332) will put you in touch with your local resource.

Additional resources

Visit the NHS smoke-free site–it's very visual, with lots of interactive aids such as a money saver calculator, video diaries and more: http://smokefree.nhs.uk

Watch the following short film on the NHS choices website:

'A Smoker's Tale'—Megan is 16 and a smoker. A make-up artist transforms her appearance to demonstrate the effects that smoking will have on her body. Will the results make Megan rethink her habit?

Nicotine replacement therapy

Nicotine replacement therapy can be a useful aid in supporting people to stop smoking; it is not a miracle solution, but using some form of nicotine replacement can make success more likely. More information is available at: http://gosmokefree.nhs.uk

Product type	How it works
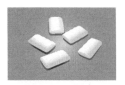 **Nicotine gum**	When you chew nicotine gum, the nicotine is absorbed through the lining of your mouth.
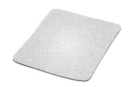 **Nicotine patches**	Nicotine patches work well for most regular smokers and can be worn around the clock (24-hour patches) or just during the day (16-hour patches).
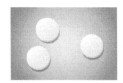 **Microtabs**	These are small tablets containing nicotine that dissolve quickly under your tongue.
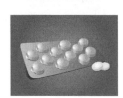 **Lozenges**	Lozenges are sucked slowly to release the nicotine and take about 20-30 minutes to dissolve.
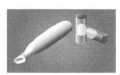 **Inhalators**	Inhalators look like a plastic cigarette. The inhalator releases nicotine vapour, which is absorbed through your mouth and throat. If you miss the 'hand-to-mouth' aspect of smoking, these may suit you.
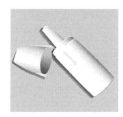 **Nicotine nasal spray**	The spray delivers a swift and effective dose of nicotine through the lining of your nose.

Other stop-smoking medicines that can help:

Product type	How it works
Zyban (bupropion hydrochloride)	Zyban is a treatment that changes the way that your body responds to nicotine. You start taking Zyban one to two weeks before you quit, and treatment usually lasts for a couple months to help you through the withdrawal cravings. It's only available on prescription, and is not available if you are pregnant.
Champix (varenicline)	Champix works by reducing your craving for a cigarette and by reducing the effects you feel if you do have a cigarette. You set a date to stop smoking, and start taking tablets one or two weeks before this date. Treatment normally lasts for 12 weeks. Champix is only available on prescription and is not available if you are pregnant. There have been reports of mental health problems in people taking Champix; however, it is very difficult to know if this is due to Champix as the act of stopping smoking itself can make people depressed. You must be 18 or over for a Champix prescription.

Additional resources

Here is an excellent local site with information to support young people who wish to stop smoking:
www.stopsmokingmanchester.co.uk/young-people.html

In addition, Action on Smoking and Health (ASH) is a campaigning public health charity that works to eliminate the harm caused by tobacco:
www.ash.org.uk

Showing the tar and gunge from a cigarette

Materials needed:

- a clear plastic bottle with a narrow neck (e.g. a small soft drink, juice or spring water bottle)
- cotton balls
- modeling clay
- a pencil
- a cigarette
- matches
- writing paper
- pencils or pens.

Perform this demonstration for students to observe because it involves matches and a cigarette.

Start the demonstration by offering a handful of students an opportunity to drop a cotton ball into the plastic bottle. Then create a ball of modeling clay and block the mouth of the bottle with it. Use a pencil to poke a hole through the modeling clay until you see the pencil tip inside the bottle; then remove the pencil.

Stick one end (the filtered end, if you are using a filtered cigarette) into the hole created in the modeling clay. Light the cigarette.

Now gently squeeze the plastic bottle to simulate breathing. Squeezing the bottle draws cigarette smoke inside the bottle the way lungs draw smoke into the body. You might let students take turns squeezing the bottle.

After pumping the bottle a dozen times or so, extinguish the cigarette. Then remove the clay plug. Ask students to observe the cotton balls in the bottom of the container.

Lead a discussion with the following questions: What happened? How do the cotton balls look? Why do they look that way? How does this demonstration show the potential effects of smoking on the body?

Additional resources

Useful websites with interactive games and quizzes:
www.safceducation.com/games/smokinggame.htm
Dodge the cigarettes and kick the football
www.roycastle.org/kats/go_games.htm
Click 'go interactive' to get started

ALCOHOL

Alcohol doesn't always attract the attention that smoking and illicit drug use do, although the consequences of alcohol abuse can be devastating. There are arguments that certain alcoholic drinks in moderation can have health benefits, but on the whole drinking when young puts unnecessary pressure on the liver, can influence decision-making and impairs thinking processes, which can have dire consequences—particularly when driving.

As with smoking, talk openly with the young people you come into contact with about alcohol. A specific session focusing on alcohol's physical and social effects will always be useful. In addition, ensure visual information is available to young people that will reinforce these health messages constantly. For example, in one of my health drop-ins, I have the posters that accompany the recent NHS advertising campaign. They display a young man who thinks he is a superhero (fuelled by alcohol) and climbs some scaffolding to try to get a girl's balloon, only to fall to his death. It always gets comments from the young people who drop in and provides a good discussion starting point.

Alcohol Statistics

1. Most young people drink.
Over 80% of 11 to 16 year olds have tried alcohol. For a quarter of those surveyed, this means having 'a few sips'.

2. Young people are drinking more.
Among young people who drink, the amount consumed has doubled since 1990 to 10 units a week. The mean consumption among 15-year-old boys who drink is nearly 12 units a week, with nine units per week for girls.

3. Young people are drinking more regularly.
The proportion of 11 to 15 year olds drinking alcohol at least once a week has risen to 24% in 2000.

4. Greater numbers are binge drinking and regularly getting drunk.
Fifteen and 16 year olds in the UK are more likely to get drunk or binge drink than most of their European counterparts, with almost a third binge drinking three or more times a month.

5. Drinking starts when children are in primary school.

Just under 5% of eight year olds have consumed a whole alcoholic drink. Fourteen per cent of girls and 21% of boys aged 10 and 11 drink each week. By the age of 13, drinkers outnumber those who don't drink. Over half of 14 and 15 year olds drink each week.

Source: *Wired for health.* Previously available at: www.wiredforhealth.gov.uk

Alcohol: the risks

- Liver damage (e.g. fatty liver, alcoholic hepatitis and cirrhosis).
- Cancer (e.g. of the mouth, larynx, pharynx and oesophagus, liver, stomach, colon and rectum and possibly breast).
- Heart disease and high blood pressure, because alcohol raises blood pressure.
- Problems with the digestive system (e.g. inflammation of the stomach lining, irritating ulcers, damage to the pancreas).
- Psychiatric disorders—Heavy drinking is closely linked with mental health problems, including clinical depression and suicide. Up to one third of young suicides had drunk alcohol at the time of death. The rise in teenage male suicide rates has been attributed to a rise in alcohol consumption.
- Reproductive problems—In men, temporary impotence and longer-term loss of potency, shrinking testes and penis and reduced sperm count.
- In women, the menstrual cycle can be disrupted, plus alcohol may increase the risk of miscarriage, can result in low birth weight babies, birth defects and foetal alcohol syndrome.
- Alcohol dependence.
- Alcohol contributes to an estimated 30,000 deaths each year, including accidents, suicides and a whole range of diseases.

Strength of alcoholic drinks

All alcoholic drinks contain pure alcohol (ethanol) in varying amounts. One way of comparing the amount of alcohol in different types of drink is by using 'units'. Each of the following contains **one unit**:

A small glass of wine = 1 UNIT

A 25 mL measure of spirit = 1 UNIT

A half pint of ordinary strength lager/beer/cider = 1 UNIT

It takes about an hour for the adult body to get rid of one unit of alcohol. This may be slower in young people.

Drink quantity units

Drink	Quantity	Units
Wine	125 mL glass	1.5
	175 mL glass	2
	75 cL bottle	6.8–7.5
	75 cL bottle	8–9
	50 mL sherry, port, Madeira, vermouth, martini	1
Lager/beer/cider	330 mL bottle	1.5
	440 mL can	2
	440 mL can	3.5–4
	500 mL can	2–2.5
	500 mL can	4–4.5
	440 mL can of low-alcohol beer	0.5
Spirits	25 mL measure	1
'Alcopops'	300 mL bottle	1.3–2
	20 cL bottle	2.7

The sensible drinking benchmarks for adults are:
- three to four units a day for men
- two to three units a day for women.

'Binge drinking' is when on one occasion men drink more than eight units and women drink more than six. No guidelines exist for children or young people's drinking. For the under-18s, 'binge-drinking' often means drinking to intoxication. Source: www.wiredforhealth.gov.uk

I have included a handout on calculating units as well as an Internet link (*see* the following box). Whilst it can be useful for young people to fully realise the amount of units they may be drinking, stress that there is no number of units that is OK—any amount of alcohol will impair decision-making ability and slow reaction times.

Additional resources

Check out the unit calculator at this link:
www.drinkaware.co.uk/tips-and-tools/drink-diary

Explore the group's existing knowledge of alcohol and the consequences of use.
Brainstorm different alcoholic drinks and explore any myths that arise.
    Brainstorm what/who influences alcohol use (e.g. friends, family, advertising, etc.).
    Brainstorm what the consequences of alcohol use could be.

Demonstrate the concentration of alcohol in different types of alcoholic drinks
Gather a shot, wine, half pint and pint glass. Put the same amount of food dye in each glass and fill each with water. Ask which is the most potent drink.

Demonstrate how alcohol can affect vision and ability
Get some beer goggles, a condom and a condom demonstrator. Let a volunteer attempt to accurately put the condom on the demonstrator. For younger participants, tying shoe laces or doing up shirt buttons can similarly demonstrate the point.

ILLEGAL DRUGS

There has been some reduction in drug use by young people in recent years. In 2006, 24% of pupils said they had used drugs, and 17% had taken drugs in the last year (an overall decrease from 13% in 2001). Five per cent of pupils had sniffed glue or other volatile substances in the last year, and 4% had taken poppers. Other drugs had been taken by less than 2% of pupils in the last year. The proportion of pupils who had taken any class A drugs in the last year had stayed at around 4% since 2001.[1]

Having said all that, we need to maintain work in drug awareness and prevention. There is much debate regarding drugs and legality in this country; whilst it might seem that government bodies can't seem to make up their minds on whether a drug is 'safe' or not, the regular coverage in the news and debate in parliament is a good thing, making people question assumptions and examine current evidence.

Use the following news item to prompt discussion on the influencing factors on how a drug is classified and how potential harm is perceived.

The government's drug adviser has accused ministers of being influenced by politics after they rejected his recommendation to reclassify ecstasy.

In February 2009 Professor David Nutt recommended the drug should be downgraded from Class A to Class B. The Home Office rejected the council's recommendation saying it was unpredictable and could kill. Professor Nutt caused controversy previously when he likened the dangers of ecstasy use and horse-riding. Some felt he was trivialising the dangers of the drug.

The advisory council reviewed the latest evidence on ecstasy and held a ballot; the majority voted to recommend moving the drug to Class B. The advisers' view is that ecstasy is not as harmful as other Class A drugs and causes far fewer deaths. It says ecstasy use has no significant impact on short-term memory loss and finds little evidence to link ecstasy to criminal behaviour. But it did call for further research into the effects of taking ecstasy, particularly on younger users.

The council's report found that over the past 10 years, deaths in which ecstasy was implicated averaged between 33 and 50 per year, while deaths where it was considered the sole drug responsible averaged between 10 to 17 per year (horse riding causes about 10 deaths a year).

Deaths from ecstasy are caused by organ failure from overheating or the effects of drinking too much water.

Drug classification

Illegal drugs are put into three controlled-drug categories: A, B and C. Class A drugs are thought to be the most dangerous and carry the most severe penalties; class C drugs are thought to be the least dangerous and carry less severe penalties.

Misuse of Drugs Act

The Misuse of Drugs Act is the main piece of legislation covering drugs and categorises drugs as class A, B and C.

These drugs are termed as controlled substances, and Class A drugs are those considered to be the most harmful.

Offences under the Act include:
* possession of a controlled substance unlawfully
* possession of a controlled substance with intent to supply it
* supplying or offering to supply a controlled drug (even where no charge is made for the drug)
* allowing premises you occupy or manage to be used unlawfully for the purpose of producing or supplying controlled drugs.

Drug trafficking (supply) attracts serious punishment, including life imprisonment for class A offences.

To enforce this law, the police have special powers to stop, detain and search people on 'reasonable suspicion' that they are in possession of a controlled drug.

Classification under the Act

Class A drugs

Include: Ecstasy, LSD, heroin, cocaine, crack, magic mushrooms, methamphetamine (crystal meth), other amphetamines if prepared for injection

Penalties for possession: Up to seven years in prison or an unlimited fine. Or both.

Penalties for dealing: Up to life in prison or an unlimited fine. Or both.

Class B drugs

Include: Cannabis, amphetamines, methylphenidate (Ritalin), pholcodine

Penalties for possession: Up to five years in prison or an unlimited fine. Or both.

Penalties for dealing: Up to 14 years in prison or an unlimited fine. Or both.

Class C drugs

Include: Tranquilisers, some painkillers, gamma-hydroxybutyrate (GHB), ketamine

Penalties for possession: Up to two years in prison or an unlimited fine. Or both.

Penalties for dealing: Up to 14 years in prison or an unlimited fine. Or both.

Source: http://drugs.homeoffice.gov.uk/drugs

DRUG INFORMATION

This information draws on the excellent drug pack resource by FRANK. It is an easy-read information pack that explores what drugs are—i.e. medicinal as well as recreational—the different reasons people use drugs and the range of reactions you could have to drugs. It contains useful fact sheets and is text light with plenty of images making it useful for a wide range of abilities.

Additional resources

The information is also available on the FRANK website at: www.talktofrank.com

Caffeine

- Stimulant
- Legal
- **Caffeine can be found in:** tea, coffee, energy drinks, cola, chocolate, ProPlus caffeine tablets

Alcohol

- Depressant
- It is legal for anyone who is 18 years old or more to buy alcohol
- Limits—women should have no more than 3 drinks a day, men no more than 4

Consequences:
Drinking too much can lead to taking risks or doing things you may regret later, having accidents, vomiting, not being aware of what you have done.
Drinking alcohol when you are pregnant could harm the baby.
It may also cause weight gain, because there are many calories in alcohol.
You may also experience increased blood pressure, liver damage, dehydration, stomach ulcers, diarrhoea, poor fertility.

Tobacco

- Stimulant
- It is illegal to sell tobacco to anyone under the age of 18

What is it?
The drug is the nicotine, which is very addictive

How does it make you feel?
People say smoking makes them feel more relaxed and helps them to concentrate

Consequences:
Smoking can cause serious lung problems, increased illness, heart problems, foetal harm if used during pregnancy, plus it can adversely effect diabetes.
Passive smoking (breathing in other people's smoke) can cause problems like asthma and cancers. It makes your skin look older; causes infertility.

Cocaine

- Stimulant
- Illegal
- Classification: Class A
- Other names: Coke, snow, Charlie

What is it?

Bitter white powder that comes from a plant that can be mixed with other things

How does it make you feel?

Energised, anxious and paranoid, confident and talkative, hot; initially highly sexed, then disinterested in sex

Consequences:

Worsens asthma, epilepsy, anxiety, depression; causes overconfidence—it may make you do things you later regret; using it when pregnant could harm the baby; damages the septum in the nose; can worsen mental health problems; can give you a heart attack (it speeds up the heart); causes liver damage; stops you from feeling hungry.

Crack

- Stimulant
- Illegal
- Classification: Class A
- Other names: Rocks, wash, stones, base, freebase

What is it?

A drug made from cocaine

How does it make you feel?

Strong, confident and chatty, energised, sick, anxious, paranoid; initially highly sexed, then disinterested in sex; the effects are stronger than cocaine

Consequences:

Worsens asthma, epilepsy, high blood pressure, anxiety, depression, heart problems; smoking it can damage lungs; causes liver damage; hallucinations; chest pain—speeds up heart; using it when pregnant could harm the baby.

It is very expensive; addicts may get involved in crime to get money to pay for it.

Ecstasy

- Depressant
- Illegal
- Classification: Class A
- Other names: E, Mitsubishis, hearts, doves

What is it?
Methylenedioxymethamphetamine, a semi-synthetic member of the amphetamine class of psychoactive drugs

How does it make you feel?
An initial rush, confusion, frightened, chatty, friendly, happy, hot and sweaty, wanting to dance, sick

Consequences:
It can worsen asthma, epilepsy, high blood pressure, anxiety, depression, heart problems (your heart beats faster), low mood a few days after taking, liver damage, poor kidney function.

Heroin

- Depressant
- Illegal
- Classification: Class A
- Other names: Smack, scag, H, horse

What is it?
A strong painkiller that can be mixed with other things

How does it make you feel?
Relaxed, safe, content, dreamy and sleepy, sick

Consequences:
Can worsen asthma, cause low blood pressure and depression. Makes skin itchy and sweaty; smoking heroin can cause lung damage, respiratory arrest, constipation, vein damage (through injecting) and slow or stop your heartbeat—resulting in death. Possible hepatitis/HIV from sharing needles.
It's very expensive; addicts may get involved in crime to pay for it.

Khat

- Stimulant
- Legal
- Other names: Quat, qat, qaadka, chat

What is it?
A leaf that you chew

How does it make you feel?
Alert and chatty, relaxed, stops you from feeling hungry. If used a lot, you can find it hard to sleep, feel anxious, feel angry, become violent

Consequences:
Can make mental health problems worse; can give you heart problems; can give you problems with sex.

LSD

- Hallucinogen
- Illegal
- Classification: Class A

What is it?
Lysergic acid diethylamide, semisynthetic psychedelic drug

Other names:
Acid, blotter, trips, micro dot, smilies, tabs

How does it make you feel?
Might see bright colours or patterns, may be frightened, people and things may look or sound different, you may not know where you are

Consequences:
Can make existing depression or anxiety worse; trips are unpredictable—good or bad—usually last around 12 hours but can be longer; can't stop it once it starts; may see flashbacks, another trip a long time after taking the drug.
It is not addictive but may cause accidents.

Magic mushrooms

- Hallucinogen
- Illegal and legal—It is not illegal to pick, have or take some sorts of magic mushrooms if they are raw, but it is illegal to dry or use some magic mushrooms in cooking or to make tea

What is it?
Psilocybin mushrooms

Other names:
Liberties, mushies, liberty cap, psilocybin, fly agaric

How do they make you feel?
Giggly, sick, confident, frightened—people and things may look or sound different, you might not know where you are

Consequences
Can make existing problems such as depression or anxiety worse; a magic mushroom trip last up to 10 hours, and you can't stop a trip once it has started; not all mushrooms are magic mushrooms, if you pick or take the wrong sort of mushrooms you could be poisoned; they may give you convulsions or flashbacks (you may have another trip a long time after taking the drug).

Poppers

- Stimulant
- Legal to buy and to have

What is it?
Direct, concentrated inhalation of amyl nitrite and the other light alkyl nitrites leading to a non-specific relaxation of smooth muscle, leading to relaxing effects in the heart and circulatory system; it is a strong-smelling liquid, sniffed from a small bottle

Other names:
Amyl nitrite, rush, liquid gold

How do they make you feel?
Full of energy, sexy, sick, dizzy, hot

Consequences:
Can make existing conditions worse: heart problems, breathing problems, anaemia, glaucoma; can kill you if swallowed, can burn skin, can give you headache and sores around mouth and nose, can stop you from getting an erection; the effects last about two minutes.

Solvents

- Depressants
- Legal
- Illegal to sell to under 18s

How can they make you feel?

Sick, dizzy, give you a headache, see or hear people that aren't there

Consequences:

Can make existing conditions worse, e.g. heart problems, blood pressure problems, epilepsy; memory loss; sores around mouth and nose; can make heart stop (death); kidney damage; liver damage; respiratory arrest. You could also pass out, choke and die.

Speed

- Stimulant
- Illegal
- Classification: Class B

What is it?

White or pink powder or tablets

Other names:

Amphetamine sulphate, sulphate, whiz, billy, uppers

How does it make you feel?

Lively or full of energy, chatty and confident, anxious, irritable and restless; afterwards: tired and depressed

Consequences:

Can make existing conditions worse: diabetes, high blood pressure, epilepsy, depression, anxiety, heart problems; makes your heart beat faster; snorting speed can damage the inside of your nose; can give you diarrhoea or cause dehydration. If you use speed when pregnant, it can harm the baby.

Anabolic steroids

- This is a class of steroid hormones related to the hormone testosterone. Anabolic steroids increase protein synthesis within cells, which results in the build up of cellular tissue (anabolism), especially in muscles. Anabolic steroids also have androgenic and virilizing properties, including the development and maintenance of masculine characteristics such as the growth of the vocal cords and body hair
- It is legal to have steroids for your own use, but it is illegal to give or sell steroids to others
- Classification: Class C, to be sold only by pharmacists with a doctor's prescription

What are they?

Medicines used to treat muscle weakness and anaemia. Can be tablets or liquid for injecting. Some people use steroids to make their muscles bigger

How do they make you feel?

Aggressive and moody; you may do things you might regret, e.g. get into fights; may have difficulty sleeping

Consequences:

Women who use steroids may: Get a deeper voice, go bald, grow hair on their face and chest, find their breasts get smaller, have period problems and put on weight *Men who use steroids might:* Go bald, grow breasts, put on weight and not be able to get an erection. They can make existing conditions worse, e.g. heart and blood pressure problems; could cause anxiety, depression; increase your chances of a stroke; could also cause bad spots; liver problems; smelly breath; heart attacks and heart disease or kidney disease.

Tranquillisers

- Depressant
- Not illegal on prescription, but illegal to give or sell to others
- Other names: Benzos, vallies, mazzies, moggies, downers
- Classification: Class C

What are they?
Prescribed medicine; strong tranquillisers used to treat mental health problems

How do they make you feel?
Relaxed and sleepy; forgetful

Consequences:
Addiction; withdrawal symptoms; the more you take the less they work; they can slow and even stop your heart beating; it is dangerous to operate machinery, e.g. drive a car, when using tranquillisers.

Cannabis

- Depressant
- Illegal
- Classification: Class B

Other names:
Grass, dope, puff, hash, pot, spliff, ganja, blow, weed, draw, skunk

What is it?
A drug taken from a plant

How does it make you feel?
Relaxed, sleepy, depressed, paranoid, giggly, hungry, confused, anxious

Consequences:
Can make existing conditions worse, e.g. heart problems, high blood pressure, asthma, depression, anxiety; it can cause lung damage (if smoked), memory problems, heart problems, infertility and digestive problems. Using when pregnant can harm the baby.

	This website can help you assess your cannabis use, its impact on your life and how to make changes if you want to: www.knowcannabis.org.uk

Get in touch with your local drug action team and ask a representative to come and speak to your group.

DRUG-ASSISTED SEXUAL ASSAULT

Drug-assisted sexual assault—or drug rape, as it is more commonly known—can be defined as the administering of a drug against an individual's wishes, or without his/her knowledge, which incapacitates or disorientates the individual with the intention of carrying out a sexual assault.

Research has shown that in over 50% of drug rape cases, the drug was administered through alcohol and 70% of attackers were known to their victims in some way.

Most instances of drug rape occur as a result of victims being in pubs and clubs, where drinking alcohol, socialising, and the hustle and bustle of the place can allow the unnoticed administration of a drug into a drink . However, other settings—such as homes, hotels, house parties, university campuses and offices—have been the scene for drug rape assaults. In addition, drug rape is not a crime exclusively perpetrated on women.

The following handout can support an informal discussion on what drug-assisted assault/rape is and what action a young person can take to avoid this situation, and in the unfortunate circumstance where it does occur, what a victim can do after the assault.

Drug-assisted rape—the facts:

* the most commonly used rape drug is alcohol
* victims are most likely to be targeted in pubs and clubs.

The rapist …
* May deliberately set out to 'spike' drinks, or may be an opportunist who takes advantage of someone who is already drunk or drugged.
* Already knows their victim in over 50% of cases.
* Is likely to work with an accomplice or gang, sometimes including women.

The victim …
* Can be male or female.
* Has memories of the attack in over 80% of cases.
* Is often a student (in up to 30% of drug rapes).

Prevention

- If you're going out drinking, remember that alcohol can affect your actions and reactions. Be careful.
- Do not accept drinks from anyone you don't know or trust, and don't share or taste other people's drinks.
- Buy bottled drinks and keep your thumb over the top when you're not drinking.
- Never leave your drink unattended.
- If you return to your drink and it has been topped up, moved, or it looks different in any way, don't drink from it again.
- Be aware that soft drinks, tea, coffee and hot chocolate can be spiked too.
- Look out for your friends; keep an eye on their drinks. If you think a drink has been spiked, get your friend out of the situation as fast as possible.

If you think you've been spiked:

- if you feel unwell, extremely drunk, or sleepy after only one or two drinks, get help straight away. You do not have much time
- ask a trusted friend for help. Failing that, go straight to the pub owner or security staff
- wherever possible DO NOT accept help from strangers or people you would not normally trust.

If you have been raped, or think you may have been:

- don't be scared to report the incident to the police, even if you are a recreational drug user, or have few or no memories of the attack. The sooner it is reported, the greater the likelihood of the offender being brought to justice
- you will probably be suffering from trauma, and should seek medical attention and support, even if you do not want to report the attack to the police
- most drugs leave the body in less than 72 hours, so try not to urinate until you have had a medical examination, or keep a sample of your urine
- if your clothes have vomit on them, it may contain whatever drug was used, and they should be kept as evidence.

Source previously available at: www.thesite.org/travelandfreetime/goingout/survival/spikeddrinks

Drugs and the law—activity

Brainstorm all the drugs you can think of, and ask the group whether each is legal or illegal.

You could do this with words written on sheets at either end of the room. Ask young people to place themselves where they feel the drug fits.

Discussion prompts:
- drugs that are legal for some and not for others, e.g. tobacco, alcohol
- drugs that are legal to buy but can be misused, e.g. poppers and solvents
- drugs that are legal but illegal if used in a certain way, e.g. steroids
- drugs that are clearly illegal, and whether they agree and why.

The effects of drugs

Split each group into three. Have all the drug names on slips of paper. Give each group an 'effect' stimulants, hallucinogens or depressants—and ask groups to identify which drugs fall into their 'effect' category.

Give each participant one or two drugs that he or she could identify as a stimulant, hallucinogen or depressant with the whole group.

Definitions:
- stimulants—Drugs that speed you up
- hallucinogens—Make you see and hear things that are not there
- depressants—Drugs that slow you down.

Examples:
- stimulants—Caffeine, cocaine, crack, ecstasy, khat, poppers, speed, steroids, tobacco
- hallucinogens—Cannabis, ecstasy, LSD, magic mushrooms
- depressants—Alcohol, heroin, solvents, tranquillisers.

Classification

Using the classification handout, ask the group to classify the following drugs:

• Cocaine	A
• Nicotine	NIL
• Caffeine	NIL
• LSD	A
• Magic mushrooms	A
• Ecstasy	A
• Benzodiazepines	C
• Heroin	A
• Anabolic steroids	NIL
• Amphetamine	B
• Cannabis	B
• Solvents (volatile substances)	NIL
• Amyl nitrites (poppers)	NIL
• Alcohol	NIL
• Crack	A

CLASSIFICATION

• Cocaine	
• Nicotine	
• Caffeine	
• LSD	
• Magic mushrooms	
• Ecstasy	
• Benzodiazepines	
• Heroin	
• Anabolic steroids	
• Amphetamine	
• Cannabis	
• Solvents (volatile substances)	
• Amyl nitrites (poppers)	
• Alcohol	
• Crack	

REFERENCE

1. The Information Centre. Smoking, drinking and drug use among young people in England in 2006. Available at: www.ic.nhs.uk/pubs/sdd06fullreport (Accessed December 2010).

CHAPTER 7

Consent, confidentiality and the law

This chapter looks at the ethical and legal issues surrounding work with young people. It will examine the issue of consent; its definition, the debate surrounding the age of consent and what the law says on underage consensual sexual intercourse. Child protection policy and procedure is summarised and the dilemma between maintaining confidentiality and child protection examined.

Consent

The definition of consent is to permit, approve, agree or yield. When thinking about the field of medical care, the area of young people and consent to treatment has raised much debate. Whether a young person is competent to consent to treatment causes many dilemmas for professionals involved in their care. If the child is under 18, and legally a minor, the parent is, in theory, responsible for the young person and should be involved in any decision. However, young people under 16 are legally able to consent to or refuse treatment provided the health professional has assessed their understanding of the procedure and any possible consequences. The Human Rights Act 1998 and the UN Convention on the Rights of the Child, to which the UK is a signatory, states that the wishes of a young person must be taken into account when considering their best interests. The Children Act 1989 gave children the authority to consent to and refuse treatment.

Consent to sexual activity

Professionals using this resource are probably working with teenagers and may have concerns about the legalities of sexual activity under the age of 16. The legal age for a sexual relationship is 16, so any young person under 16 engaging in sexual intercourse is acting illegally. However, as we know from looking at how young people develop physically, mentally and socially, they don't automatically become competent to make reasoned decisions on their 16th birthday!

The ability to reason and understand the consequences of a course of action is a gradual process and can begin well before the age of 16. The law does acknowledge this. It is recognised that children and young people have rights regarding what happens to their bodies and can have the ability to make a reasoned and rational decision.

For those working in a general capacity with young people, relationships and sexual activity will be a consideration; is the young person in an appropriate relationship? How can the professional support the person's emerging sexuality whilst maintaining safety and remaining within the law? As previously mentioned, in England the legal age for heterosexual and homosexual intercourse is 16 years. However, although not legal, children between the ages of 13 and 15 are considered able to consent to sexual intercourse. Children below the age of 13 are deemed legally incompetent to consent to sexual activity and as such all sexual intercourse would be considered non-consensual.

Fraser competency

There was some confusion in the early 80s regarding issuing contraceptives to girls under 16 as to whether parents should be involved. In 1974, the Department of Health and Social Security (DHSS) issued a memo of guidance to doctors advising that contraceptive advice could be given to girls aged under 16 without informing their parents and that they should always ask the girl's permission to tell her parents. However, the memo was followed up in 1980 by an adage: the need to persuade the girl to involve the parents or guardian and that the decision to involve the parents or not lay with the clinician. Naturally the way this was interpreted varied widely between clinicians. Some carried on as before, advising and issuing contraception to under 16s, encouraging the young woman to talk to her parents; other young people were told they would have to bring their parents to the appointment. As a result, young people felt that confidential advice and treatment was not universally available to under 16s.

Eventually following one mother's (Victoria Gillick) unsuccessful attempt to gain assurance that her daughters would not be provided with contraceptive advice or treatment without her consent through the law courts, clearer and more explicit guidelines were produced. These guidelines made clear that health professionals could provide contraceptive advice and treatment to young people, without informing their parents, provided that certain conditions were met. These conditions are called the Fraser Guidelines, named after the judge who presided over the case. Each time a young person consults for treatment, an assessment should be made of their competence to consent and deemed 'Gillick competent'.

This judgement referred specifically to doctors but it is considered to apply to other health professionals working with young people. It may also be interpreted as covering youth workers and health promotion workers who may be giving contraceptive advice and condoms to young people under 16, but this has not been tested in court.

The Fraser Guidelines:

Health professionals are able to provide contraceptive advice and treatment to under 16s as long as the following conditions are met:
- the young person understands the professional's advice
- the young person is encouraged to inform their parents
- the young person is likely to begin, or to continue having, sexual intercourse with or without contraceptive treatment
- unless the young person receives contraceptive treatment, his or her physical or mental health, or both, are likely to suffer
- the young person's best interests require him or her to receive contraceptive advice or treatment with or without parental consent.

Although these criteria specifically refer to contraception, the principles are deemed to apply to other treatments, including abortion.

Similar provision is made in Scotland by the Age of Legal Capacity (Scotland) Act 1991. In Northern Ireland, although separate legislation applies, what was then the Department of Health and Social Services Northern Ireland stated that there was no reason to suppose that the House of Lords' decision would not be followed by the Northern Ireland Courts.

Consent and young people with learning difficulties

Young people with learning difficulties should have the same access to services as other young people. Professionals working with this group need to be creative when presenting information to young people with learning difficulties so they can understand their options and the consequences of choices to the best of their ability. This may involve presenting the information pictorially, or using other forms of communication aids, e.g. the use of Makaton symbols or an advocate.

Books Beyond Words

Picture books are available from the Royal College of Psychology for adults and adolescents who cannot read or who have difficulty reading. They provide information and address the emotional aspects of difficult events. Each book actively addresses the problems of understanding that people with learning and communication difficulties experience.

The stories are told through colour pictures that include mime and body language to communicate simple, explicit messages. These help 'readers' to cope with emotions and events such as going to the doctor, bereavement, sexual abuse and depression.
www.rcpsych.ac.uk/publications/booksbeyondwords/bbwtitlesa-z.aspx

Access to health services by under 16s

Despite the Fraser Guidelines being in existence for nearly 20 years, there are still health professionals who will not see an unaccompanied child under 16 years of age; this can lead to young people not being able to access the services and advice they require.

The 'You're Welcome' criteria, which sets out how a service can become young-people friendly and is spearheaded by the government, is raising the profile of young people's needs; however, a young person may need support in accessing appropriate services.

You're Welcome

All young people are entitled to receive appropriate health care wherever they access it. The You're Welcome quality criteria lay out principles that will help health services—both in the community and in hospitals—to 'get it right' and become young-people friendly.

The quality criteria cover 10 topic areas:
- accessibility
- publicity
- confidentiality and consent
- the environment
- staff training, skills, attitudes and values
- joined-up working
- monitoring and evaluation, and involvement of young people
- health issues for adolescents
- sexual and reproductive health services
- child and adolescent mental health services (CAMHS).

For more information, *see* the following link:
www.dh.gov.uk/en/Publicationsandstatistics/Publications/PublicationsPolicyAndGuidance/DH_073586

AGE OF CONSENT: DEBATE

Debate surrounding the age of consent presents extreme viewpoints. Some feel that the age should be lowered to reflect current sexual activity of young people; some feel that it is fine as it is, reflecting an age between childhood and adulthood; some feel that it should be raised to protect young people from unwanted pregnancy and STIs; some feel that it should be abolished so that sexuality and sex is decriminalised.

The following quotes show what young people think of the age of consent:

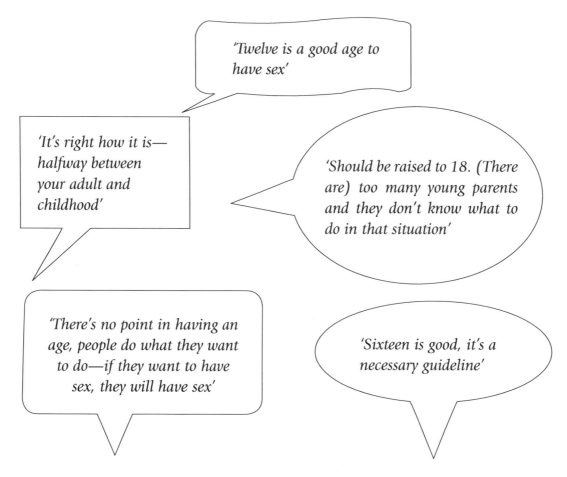

Source: Channel 4. *Sex before 16: where the law is failing*. Available through the British Film Institute archives at: http://ftvdb.bfi.org.uk/sift/title/783550?view=synopsis (Accessed 2003).

Who decides the age of consent?

Campaigners in the 1860s, when the age of consent stood at 12, fought to stop young girls being sold to brothels. They succeeded in getting parliament to raise the age to 13. This was then raised to 16 in 1885 when an account was published in a journal of how easy it was to purchase a 13 year old for prostitution.

Should the age of consent be lowered?

Some teenagers are having sexual experiences long before the legal age of consent, and the law should recognise this to be able to give the proper advice and support to prevent diseases, unwanted pregnancies and abuse. For example, if 14 year olds are not legally allowed to have sex, it is very difficult to discuss it with them at school. On the whole, young people do not pay any heed to the law when contemplating sexual relations:

'If you feel the time is right…I don't think anyone should be stopped'

'It's nature; you can't have a law against nature'

'The law isn't relevant to me; when I've found someone and I'm confident to lose my virginity, I'm not going to think about the law'

Source: Channel 4. *Sex before 16: where the law is failing.* Available through the British Film Institute archives at: http://ftvdb.bfi.org.uk/sift/title/783550?view=synopsis (Accessed 2003).

Some critics argue that today's culture is becoming increasingly sex obsessed—through adverts, TV and provocative clothing—and this is pressurising teenagers to try to keep up with what they perceive to be the correct way to behave by being sexually active. People of this opinion say that the last thing that we should be doing is lowering the age of consent to send yet another message that young people are expected to have sex early.

Many believe that lowering the age of sexual consent will in fact encourage young people to have sex earlier and place them at greater risk of diseases, unwanted pregnancies and abuse.

This is not necessarily the case. Some countries have a lower age of consent and yet a higher age of first intercourse. For example, in Spain the age of consent is 13 and average age of first sex is 19 for girls and 18 for boys; in Los Angeles in America the age of consent is 18 and age of first sex is 17; and in Chile the age of consent is 12 and age of first sex is 15 for girls and 14 for boys. For a better idea of what influences the age at which first sexual intercourse occurs, we would need to examine how the culture of each country influences sexual behaviour and how it compares to Great Britain rather than simply look to the law.

In addition, apparent recent increases in teen sexual activity do not necessarily mean that any more people are having sex earlier than they did in previous generations, just that we are more honest and efficient at recording data, and society has a more open attitude to young people's sexuality. We also expect more from young people before settling into a relationship and we look to the possible consequences of relationships, e.g. the sacrifice of academic achievements or financial security.

Should the age of consent be raised?

Another viewpoint is that if the age of consent is left at 16 or raised it will mean that young people may receive the message that they are doing something wrong and will not feel confident to seek sexual health and contraceptive advice. As it stands at the moment it could be said that the law is hypocritical, setting the age of consent at 16 yet making contraception available to under 16s: ensuring that young people break the law safely! One way to deal with this reality, and to continue current positive trends such as a decline in unwanted teenage pregnancies, is to legally recognise that teenagers are having sex at a younger age. Then the issue is in the open, and young people will feel free to seek advice, counselling and direction in their relationships.

Should there be an age of consent at all?

Setting an age of consent is considered by some as arbitrary; a young person may be physically mature but not necessarily emotionally ready for a sexual relationship. An age of consent is a barrier that, if removed, gives young people freedom to talk, seek advice and take responsibility for their own actions.

One proposal would be to set the age of consent at the border between childhood and adolescence and not between adolescence and adulthood. This would maintain childhood innocence whilst supporting consensual teenage experimentation. Interestingly, no country has an age of consent lower than 12, and no country has abolished the age of consent.

Whatever the conclusion, it is essential that the focus should shift towards education and communication to support young people in making informed choices, rather then legislation. Also there should be an effective and workable definition of consent to protect young people in their emerging sexuality.

The age of consent debate
- What do you think the age of consent should be? Why?
- Present where the age of consent in this country has come from.
- Present a range of ages of consent in different countries and discuss the average age of first sexual intercourse in relation to age of consent.
- Explore the possible reasons for different outcomes in different areas.
- Present the legalities in this country, including the Fraser Guidelines.

Scenario

Discuss the following scenario with your group:

An interview with five live listeners concerning John and Pat, who are mum and dad to 16-year-old Lee.

'Lee is sleeping with his 13-year-old girlfriend, and Lee's mum and dad are at their wits' end. They are petrified their son is going to ruin his and the young girl's life. They have actually been to the police to report their son **and** to social services—neither of whom believe the case is a priority. They got in touch with us because having done all they feel they **can** do, they would appreciate your advice. What should they do?'

As presented on the Victoria Derbyshire show on 5 Live (2 April 2009)

Some of the comments presented on the show's blog included the following comments. These could be use to prompt further debate.

'Why do they expect everyone else to sort out THEIR SON?! Wondering why he won't take responsibility for his own actions? Look at his role models!'

'Two points: Children don't listen to their parents, and this isn't a new thing. Kids have done what they wanted to for decades without taking authority into the equation.

Second, underage sex isn't new either. My wife lost her virginity at 14 and that was the 70s. I don't doubt that sex in early teens has been going on since time immemorial.

Yes, parents should advise their children to wait until they are of legal age to be doing this sort of thing, but in the end if two people want to have sex then they are going to.'

'At some point they will split up; there will be people out there who will have an interest in making this girl see herself as the victim. He WILL eventually be interviewed and arrested. Her word against his and you know who they will believe as it will be politically expedient to take the girl's side.

This boy is ruining the whole of his life and the parents can see that. He will struggle to get a job as the fact that he is on the sex-offenders register will haunt him at 20, at 30, at 40 and so on.'

'Either it is illegal to have sex with a 13-year-old girl or it isn't. He is over 16, when is it OK then . . . 17, 18, 20, 22, 25 (getting worried yet?), 30, 35, 40? And then why not 12, 11, 10 . . . really worried now, are you?'

'One thing that isn't being discussed here is the girl and the parents of the girl. If they are aware of this going on, are they not neglecting her by allowing this liaison to occur? Are her parents not only morally neglecting her but legally responsible for her conduct, ... is the girl not guilty of having sex whilst below the legal age?'

THERE'S MORE TO IT THAN THE LAW . . .

Of course, consent to sexual activity doesn't simply involve whether a young person is of legal age to consent; in addition the young person should be making his or her own choice based on enjoyment and not coercion or pressure.

To make a free and voluntary choice a person must feel:

- safe
- trust
- listened to; that he or she has options, e.g. 'yes', 'no', 'not now', 'maybe later', 'never'
- respected, whatever his or her choice
- able to stop at any time.

A free and voluntary choice never involves:

- force
- threats
- coercion
- intimidation
- blackmail
- tricks
- deception or fraud.

 Discuss the following points with your group of young people to explore whether they feel able to gage whether their partner would be fully consenting to sexual activity.

How can you ensure your partner is making a free and voluntary choice to engage in sexual activity with you?

- An effective way of doing this is to focus upon each person's enjoyment. Questions aimed at finding ways to increase a person's pleasure often have questions about consent built into them. For example, 'Are you enjoying this?' 'Would you like me to continue?'
- Non-verbal cues are also important. Does the other person return your kisses and touches, or does he/she push you away or try to avoid getting closer?
- If a person does not offer verbal or physical resistance, this should not be taken to mean that they are making a free and voluntary choice. Sometimes a person can 'freeze' because they are too frightened or intimidated to show how they are feeling.
- Where there is a possibility that a person is not making a free and voluntary choice, or you are unsure, the safest and most ethical choice is to stop what you are doing and ask.
- Where a person says or indicates that they do not want to continue, or is still unclear, then the only choice is to stop.

Discuss the following scenarios in groups. Divide your group into three, give them a scenario each and ask the groups to give feedback to the wider group, inviting comments and debate.

Scenario 1

It's a great party. Lani is having a fantastic time. Feeling confident and flirtatious, she approaches Andrew, a cute guy she has had her eye on, and invites him to hook up at the end of the night. When Andrew finds Lani later, she is so drunk that she has passed out on a bed. He has sex with her anyway.

Scenario 2

Darryn's mates tease him for being a virgin. One night at the pub, they charm Tatiana, a young woman they have previously called a slut, into coming onto him. They tell her that Darryn is keen on her and that she should make a move. When Darryn refuses her advances, his mates encourage her to keep touching and stroking him. Meanwhile, they ply both of them with alcohol and ridicule Darryn, calling him 'shy' and a 'poofta' every time he pushes her away. Eventually, Darryn starts playing along with the joke, touching and stroking Tatiana in return. At the end of the night, Darryn and Tatiana stumble out the door together, very drunk. Darryn's mates presume that they are off to have sex and celebrate this as a victory for the boys having broken their friend's resolve.

Scenario 3

Ahmid's girlfriend Dahlia has finally agreed to have sex with him. They decide that Friday night is the night. After kissing and petting for a while, they start to remove each other's clothes. When Ahmid gets to Dahlia's underwear she says 'no' and shakes her head. He keeps going anyway, just to test the waters. Because she doesn't offer any more resistance, he keeps going. After all, they had an agreement. Eventually, he ends up having intercourse with her, but it's not very pleasant. Although Dahlia doesn't stop him, she's really stiff and seems uncomfortable.

The above section on consensual sex and the scenarios are adapted with thanks from: www.purplearmband.org/about.htm

Purple Armband Games are sports fixtures where teams wear purple armbands while they play. Purple Armband Games aim to empower the silent majority of men and women to speak out against violent and abusive behaviours towards women.

Abusive situations

Child sexual abuse is the sexual molestation of children by adults or older children (sexual here means any activity that leads to sexual arousal in the perpetrator). Working Together to Safeguard Children (the government guidance on child protection) describes it as:

> Forcing or enticing a child or young person to take part in sexual activities, whether or not the child is aware of what is happening. The activities may include penetrative (e.g. rape or buggery) or non-penetrative acts. They may include non-contact activities, such as involving children in looking at pornographic material or watching sexual activities, or encouraging children to behave in sexually inappropriate ways.

Estimates now state that at least one in four males and one in three females will have encountered some form of sexual abuse before reaching the age of 18.

The clearest picture we have to date of the prevalence of sexual abuse of children is the National Society for the Prevention of Cruelty to Children (NSPCC) study 'Child Maltreatment'. The study found that, contrary to stereotype, sexual abuse by a parent or caregiver is relatively rare and that sexual abuse by a relative most commonly involves a brother or stepbrother. However, a more frequent perpetrator than a relative is someone known to, but unrelated to, the child. Most interesting for this book is that the most common age to suffer abuse by a known but unrelated perpetrator is between 13 and 15, and most of the victims are girls. Very few victims told anyone at the time; if they did they were most likely to have confided in a friend, sometimes in a relative and very rarely in a professional.

As well as being traumatic for the young person at the time, the abuse can have serious psychological consequences in later life such as depression and anxiety, self-harm and even suicide.

Children who are abused sexually can be groomed and trained, the process occurring over months or years. Children may develop a pattern of adjustment to the abuse displaying characteristics such as: secrecy, helplessness, self-blame, delayed disclosure and retraction.

Additional resources

Working Together to Safeguard Children
Working Together to Safeguard Children sets out how individuals and organisations should work together to safeguard and promote the welfare of children.

This government site offers specific guidance and examples of good practice when working with young people under 18 years old. To learn more, search 'working together' at:

www.dcsf.gov.uk/everychildmatters

Internet grooming

Grooming is the process of getting to know and befriending a child with the intention of sexually abusing them. Children have it drummed into them that they shouldn't talk to or go anywhere with strangers, so paedophiles often take their time to build up a trusting relationship. Grooming doesn't have to be online, but the internet gives paedophiles the anonymity to act more freely, and access to children who are not under direct parental supervision.

In this context, therefore, grooming is the process by which a person befriends a child to gain his or her trust and to create a situation whereby the child will allow the perpetrator to have sexual contact with him or her and will not tell anyone about it. Grooming is an integral part of virtually all sexual abuse, but what concerns people about internet grooming in particular is the fear that the cycle can be speeded up. The internet enables people to be anonymous online and thus characteristics such as age and sex can be hidden. This allows for the befriending stage to occur more quickly as trust is built through the child thinking he or she is talking to someone of his or her own generation.

A report by the cyberspace research unit at the University of Central Lancashire has set out the 'grooming' process used by paedophiles to befriend children over the internet with the intention of abusing them.[1]

1. Friendship
Flattering a child into talking in a private chat room where he or she will be isolated. The child will often be asked for a non-sexual picture of him or herself.

2. Forming a relationship
Asking the child what problems he has to create the illusion of being his best friend.

3. Risk assessment
Asking the child about the location of his computer and who else has access to it in order to assess the risk of being detected.

4. Exclusivity
Building up a sense of mutual love and trust with the child, suggesting that they can discuss 'anything'.

5. Sex talk
Engaging the child in explicit conversations and requesting sexually explicit pictures from them. At this stage, the paedophile will usually try to arrange a meeting with the child.

Discuss the following script of an attempt by a paedophile to engage a young girl through an Internet chat room:

The Government's Child Exploitation and Online Protection Centre has published this edited version of how a suspected paedophile attempted to groom a 13-year-old schoolgirl through a text conversation on a social networking website. The suspected paedophile calls himself ST*R boy, the schoolgirl is Angelgurl. Translations of email slang are in brackets.

Chat Log:

ST*R boy: ASL [age, sex, location]?
Angelgurl: 13, f, Best town in the world!
ST*R boy: where's that then??
Angelgurl: Nottingham. U?
ST*R boy: m, 16, London. What u look like?
Angelgurl: I dunno! Blondey hair, short, green eyes.
ST*R boy: big t***?
Angelgurl: lol [laugh out loud]
ST*R boy: U got a webcam?:
Angelgurl: ycah
ST*R boy: Wanna play? Turn it on
Angelgurl: brb [be right back—said as the girl goes to plug in her web video camera in her room]
Angelgurl: k. bk. [ok. back] What u up 2?
ST*R boy: I'm horny J how u feelin?
Angelgurl: lets talk bout somfink else
ST*R boy: cm on angel. bet u is an angel. Turn on ur cam
Angelgurl: k. but u turn it on 1st. I am an angel really!
ST*R boy: cm on, b fun—yeah. [the girl has now turned her web camera on] That's it, that's nice. U pretty.
Angelgurl: fanks J
ST*R boy: I wanna c more—take that top off??
Angelgurl: nah! Turn ur cam on??
ST*R boy: As soon as u show me those t***!! Lol
Angelgurl: u rude
ST*R boy: whats ur mobile? I'll send u a pic.
Angelgurl: I can't give u that; my mum wud kill me.
ST*R boy: wot kind of m8 doesn't give digits?? I can't take u out if u don't give me ur numbers.

Angelgurl: my mum would be mad

ST*R boy: ur mum's neva gonna knw. What happens between us stays between us right?

Angelgurl: yea

ST*R boy: I'm gonna be dreamin bout u angel. U so sexy. Wanna touch urself for me?

Angelgurl: u rude. Stop it

ST*R boy: cum on angel—u sexy wen u angry. Be gud 2 touch u in person—im touching my **** now just looking at u.

Angelgurl: I'm gonna stop soon.

ST*R boy: cum on angel. show sum skin

Angelgurl: no

ST*R boy: I'm in Nottingham nxt wk if u fancy it? I'll show u my ****

Angelgurl: ur 2 intense—turn on ur cam so I can c who u r.

ST*R boy: it's broken—but I'll send u a pic if u give me ur mobile? How will u recognise me otherwise wen I come 2 urs??

Angelgurl: u don't knw where I am

ST*R boy: yeah I do angel. I know exactly who u r and where u r. I;m gona drive up 2 u now.

Angelgurl: How can u drive—u 16??

ST*R boy: Got my provisional

Angelgurl: u lyin?? U 2 old 4 me?

ST*R boy: nah angel. I'm perfect 4 u.

Angelgurl: I'm going now. Ur weird.

ST*R boy: I'll find u again angel—I wana chat more…

Angelgurl signs off.

Safety messages for online chat

1 Don't give out personal details, photographs, or any other information that could be used to identify you, such as information about your family, where you live or the school you go to.

2 Don't take other people at face value—they may not be what they seem.

3 Never arrange to meet someone you've only ever previously met on the internet without first telling your parents, getting their permission and taking a responsible adult with you. The first meeting should always be in a public place.

4 Always stay in the public areas of chat where there are other people around.

5 Don't open an attachment or downloaded file unless you know and trust the person who has sent it.

6 Never respond directly to anything you find disturbing—save or print it, log off, and tell an adult.

CONFIDENTIALITY

An area that all professionals encounter when working with adolescents is what degree of confidentiality can we offer them. For health professionals, confidentiality is where information between professional and client remains within the consultation. Everyone is entitled to a confidential consultation regardless of age. This can only be broken if there are child protection issues or concerns for the client or others. For teaching staff, confidentiality parameters may be different, as they are acting *in loco parentis* and have an obligation to discuss issues with parents. The main consideration is to ensure that young people are aware of the degree of confidentiality available to them before disclosure.

When asked about barriers to seeking advice regarding sexual health, concern over confidentiality is most often quoted by young people. Professionals are concerned that if there are child protection issues they cannot guarantee complete confidentiality. Young people under the age of 16 have as great a right to confidentiality as anyone. If someone under 16 is not judged mature enough to consent to treatment, the consultation itself can still remain confidential. Professionals working with young people will have a duty of confidentiality and should make themselves aware of the policy; they must not disclose anything learned from a person who has consulted or whom they have examined or treated, without that person's agreement. Confidentiality may only be broken in the most exceptional circumstances when the health, safety or welfare of the patient, or others, would be at grave risk.

There can be difficulties in providing confidential sexual health services to young people. Whilst they are entitled to the same degree of confidentiality as adults and can consent to examination and treatment if judged to be Fraser-competent, their sexual activity may be unlawful either due to their age, the age of their partner or if they are involved in prostitution. Sexual activity is particularly an issue for the under 13s. They can be judged Fraser-competent to consent to examination and treatment but are regarded as incapable of consenting to sexual activity, requiring referral to child protection services or the police.

When should information be disclosed?

Although every effort is made to give young people equal rights to confidentiality, there are certain occasions when a professional may have to consider disclosure of information to child protection services:

- when a child is sexually active under the age of 13
- when a child between the ages of 13 and 15 is having consensual sex with a partner who is more than five years older
- when there is disclosure of or suspected sexual abuse
- when the disclosure of information may be the only way to protect the client from serious harm
- when other children may potentially be at risk
- when children under 16 are involved in commercial sex work.

Naturally, a balance needs to be found between the need to protect the young person from harm and the person's right to confidentiality. The aim is to develop a relationship of trust with the young person. Each situation must be assessed individually before any decision to disclose is made.

If the young person is opposed to the requirement to break confidentiality, attempts should be made to work with him or her to make consent to disclosure acceptable. It may be possible to work with the young person over a period of time in order to obtain consent, unless there is evidence of immediate danger or risk to another child.

Professionals providing these services have to weigh up the child protection issues for these young people, whilst considering the needs and rights of the young person for confidential and appropriate medical care. If a service is not seen to be confidential, there is a risk that either it will not be accessed, or that those attending will not be honest about their age and/or sexual activity and may not disclose abuse or exploitation. This can have serious health implications and mean that abuse might go unrecognised, and the opportunity for supporting the young person and intervention would be lost.

It is always recommended to discuss any concerns you have regarding child protection with a colleague and/or line manager and document any discussions you have.

A whole-team approach

Confidentiality issues are not simply relevant for the one-to-one consultation. All staff involved in a young person's service should be aware of confidentiality issues and be aware of their professional code of confidentiality as well as the service's confidentiality policy. There needs to be a whole-team approach to confidentiality.

The contribution of all professionals to the safeguarding of children is essential. Often many professionals come into contact with a young person who is being abused. The young person may confide in a professional or the professional may get a gut feeling that something is not right. This information or feeling may not seem important on its own and the professional may think it's not significant enough to take further. However other professionals may be in a similar position and the combination of information can build a picture that will warrant an investigation.

It can be difficult to assess the significance of the information about a child, to gage its seriousness and decide what to do next. Discussion with clinicians reveals that most are comfortable dealing with disclosures of definite abuse. More often, however, they are faced with ambiguous situations. These vary from case to case and should be dealt with on an individual basis. To help identify and clarify the concern, it is helpful to discuss the situation with other members of your team or the named professional with responsibility for child protection issues in your team. Often, child protection issues are complicated with layers of concern: the immediate physical safety of the child, the psychological condition of the child (he may not think he is in an abusive situation), protection from STIs and pregnancy, etc.

Accessing support

There is a named nurse and doctor responsible for child protection within community health services and education. As they deal with child protection cases all the time, they have the ability to draw out the actual concerns for the young person and have the expertise to advise on a plan of action for the particular situation. It is possible to discuss your concerns without identifying the young person.

Social services is the central point for reporting any concerns you may have regarding a young person. It is possible to ring social services and speak informally to the duty social worker about a situation and take his or her advice on whether the concern should be formally reported. The duty social worker will ask you the name and address of the young person; this is to see if they already have a file on the child or other children in the family, and it is part of the social worker's role—to collect information and build a picture of what is happening in a family or situation.

Keeping a record

At every step, it is essential to record your concerns and what steps you have taken to take this further. Records should include objective observations, the content of discussion between yourself and the young person, and discussions with other professionals. Times and dates are crucial. These notes should be written at the time of contact or very soon afterwards to ensure accuracy of information. The notes should follow the child if he or she moves so professionals that will be coming into contact with the young person will have information on their situation and can carry on any work the multi-disciplinary team has been carrying out in your area. As professionals, we are accountable for our actions and it is only the written record that will be credible if the case should go to child protection conference or even to court.

Confidentiality and Young People Toolkit.

by RCGP and Brook (2000)

This is a resource outlining law and issues surrounding confidentiality, with copiable overheads for teaching and adaptable pro formas for use in the clinical setting.

Email: info@rcgp.org.uk
Website: www.rcgp.org.uk

What should I do?

Guidance on confidentiality for community nurses, social workers, teachers and youth workers.is available from Brook Publications.

Email: admin@brookcentres.org.uk

'Trust'

This 10-minute video designed to trigger discussion on confidentiality policy and young people.is available from the Royal College of General Practitioners. *See* previously noted contact information.

Additional resources

What to do if you're worried a child is being abused
The Department of Education has information that can help:
http://education.gov.uk/publications/standard/publicationDetail/
Page1/31981

REFERENCE

1. University of Central Lancashire: Cyberspace Research Unit. *Cyber Stalking, Abusive Cyber Sex and Online Grooming: a programme of education for teenagers.* http://new.vawnet.org/category/Documents.php?docid=526&category_id=93 (Accessed 2004).

CHAPTER 8

Relationships and sex

This chapter serves as an introduction to the area of relationships and sex. I have deliberately put the word relationships before sex, as I hope we would be encouraging young people to have a fun friendship before starting a sexual relationship. However, Sex and Relationships Education, or SRE, is what it is more commonly termed. The factual aspects of SRE tend to be easier to deal with; and the areas of contraception, STIs, pregnancy and abortion will be looked at in more detail in subsequent chapters. More difficult, yet vital, is the context of this activity, the relationship itself. How do we encourage young people to have healthy, edifying relationships?

Through example and activity we should show that there is value in being single, that there is no need to rush into having relationships, to enable young people to explore who they are before becoming part of a couple. However, it is important to recognise that being in a relationship can be positive too, if there is mutual respect. Our role here is to help young people know how to negotiate within a relationship, how to evaluate whether the relationship is good, and to be aware of what influences attitudes and sexual activity within relationships.

SRE curriculum

If you are thinking of looking at any kind of sex and relationship issues with the young people in your group, it would be a good idea to know what content, detail and context the government recommends for each age group. This way you can ensure that you are not giving inappropriate information to young people; this protects both them and you. It would also be expedient to inform parents when you are going to look at this subject, for although it can be frustrating, parents do have the right to remove their child from sex and relationship education (SRE).

The SRE curriculum for key stages three and four (secondary school level) are a useful guide for group work in youth groups.

Additional resources

National curriculum

To view the full national curriculum, visit www.nc.uk.net

Good to know

- The PSHE and Citizenship framework provides a planning tool for holistic provision of SRE.
- The biological content of sex education is laid out in the National Science Curriculum. The Education Act 1996 requires all maintained secondary schools to provide a sex education curriculum that includes teaching about HIV/AIDS and STIs.

A summary would be as follows:
- both boys and girls should be prepared for puberty
- young people need access to, and precise information about, confidential contraceptive information, advice and services
- young people need to be aware of the moral and personal dilemmas involved in abortion and know how to access a relevant agency if necessary
- young people need to be aware of the risks of STIs, including HIV, and know about prevention, diagnosis and treatment
- young people need to know not just what safer sex is and why it is important, but also how to negotiate it with a partner.

SRE is lifelong learning about sex, sexuality, emotions, relationships and sexual health. It involves acquiring accurate information, developing skills, positive values and a moral framework that will guide decision-making, judgements and behaviour. The Sex Education Forum (of the National Children's Bureau) describes sex education as having three elements: the acquisition of information; the development of social skills; and the development of moral responsibility and values. This is a good framework to bear in mind when tackling SRE in youth organisations.

SRE Policy

Schools must have an SRE, policy and it is a good idea for youth groups to have one too if they are going to tackle SRE content. This ensures that all staff and anyone who reads the policy is aware of, and assured that, the content of sessions will reflect national recommendations. The following policy is a template set out by the Healthy Schools programme and can be adapted to reflect the aims and ethos of other youth organizations.

Additional resources

Healthy schools

This is an exciting long-term initiative that promotes the link between **good health**, **behaviour** and **achievement**. Offering close support and guidance to primary care trusts, local authorities and their schools, Healthy Schools equips children and young people with the skills and knowledge to make informed health and life choices and to reach their full potential. Learn more at: www. healthyschools.gov.uk

Example Sex and Relationship Education Policy

1. Name of organisation:
Date of policy:

This policy was developed in response to Sex and Relationship Education Guidance DfES 2000, the National Teenage Pregnancy Strategy and the National Healthy Schools Programme.

2. The consultation process has involved:

Describe the consultation that has taken place, for example:

- pupil/young people's focus groups
- questionnaires to parents/carers
- any consultation with the wider community, e.g. the school nurse.

3. What is Sex and Relationship Education (SRE)?

SRE is lifelong learning about physical, sexual, moral and emotional development. It is about the understanding of the importance of stable and loving relationships, respect, love and care for family life. It involves acquiring information, developing skills and forming positive beliefs, values and attitudes.

4. Principles and values

In addition, **<Name of organisation>** believes that SRE should:

- be an integral part of the lifelong learning process, beginning in early childhood and continuing into adult life
- be an entitlement for all young people
- encourage every young person to contribute to our community and aim to support each individual as they grow and learn

- be set within this wider youth context and support family commitment and love, respect and affection, knowledge and openness. Family is a broad concept; there is not just one model, e.g. the nuclear family. It includes a variety of types of family structure, and acceptance of different approaches
- encourage young people/youth leaders to share and respect each other's views. We are aware of different approaches to sexual orientation, without promotion of any particular family structure. The important values are love, respect and care for each other
- generate an atmosphere where questions and discussion on sexual matters can take place without any stigma or embarrassment
- recognise that parents are the key people in teaching their children about sex, relationships and growing up. We aim to work in partnership with parents and young people, consulting them about the content of programmes
- recognise that the wider community has much to offer and that we aim to work in partnership with health professionals, social workers, peer educators and other mentors or advisers.

Sex and Relationship Education in this school/youth group has three main elements:

Attitudes and values
- Learning the importance of values, individual conscience and moral choices.
- Learning the value of family life, stable and loving relationships, and marriage.
- Learning about the nurture of children.
- Learning the value of respect, love and care.
- Exploring, considering and understanding moral dilemmas.
- Developing critical thinking as part of decision-making.
- Challenging myths, misconceptions and false assumptions about normal behaviour.

Personal and social skills
- Learning to manage emotions and relationships confidently and sensitively.
- Developing self-respect and empathy for others.
- Learning to make choices with an absence of prejudice.
- Developing an appreciation of the consequences of choices made.
- Managing conflict.
- Empowering young people with the skills to be able to avoid inappropriate pressures or advances (both as the exploited or the exploiter).

Knowledge and understanding

- Learning and understanding physical development at appropriate stages.
- Understanding human sexuality, reproduction, sexual health, emotions and relationships.
- Learning about contraception and the range of local and national sexual health advice, contraception and support services.
- Learning the reasons for delaying sexual activity, and the benefits to be gained from such delay.
- Avoiding unplanned pregnancy.

5. Aims

Here you should take the opportunity to highlight your aims in relation to your youth group values and ethos. Your status, e.g. school/group, will influence these aims. Below are some examples that you may wish to consider:

The aim of SRE is to provide balanced factual information about human reproduction, together with consideration of the broader emotional, ethical, religious and moral dimensions of sexual health. Our SRE programme aims to prepare students for an adult life in which they can:

- develop positive values and a moral framework that will guide their decisions, judgements and behaviour; have the confidence and self-esteem to value themselves and others and respect for individual conscience; and have the skills to judge what kind of relationship they want
- understand the consequences of their actions and behave responsibly within sexual and platonic relationships
- avoid being exploited or exploiting others or being pressured into unwanted or unprotected sex
- communicate effectively by developing appropriate terminology for sex and relationship issues
- develop awareness of their sexuality and understand human sexuality; challenge sexism and prejudice, and promote equality and diversity
- understand the arguments for delaying sexual activity
- understand the reasons for having protected sex
- have sufficient information and skills to protect themselves and their partner (if they have one) from uninvited/unwanted conceptions and sexually transmitted infections including HIV
- be aware of sources of help and acquire the skills and confidence to access confidential health advice, support and treatment if necessary
- know how the law applies to sexual relationships.

6. Organisation and content of sex and relationship education

Any SRE session may consider questions or issues that some students will find sensitive. Before embarking on these lessons, ground rules should be established, which prohibit inappropriate personal information being requested or disclosed by those taking part in the lesson. When young people ask questions, we aim to answer them honestly, within the ground rules established at the start of the sessions. When it is felt that answering a specific question would involve information at a level inappropriate to the development of the rest of the group, the question may be dealt with individually at another time.

7. Inclusion

This should be specific to the needs of your group; however, you may wish to consider the following:

Ethnic and cultural groups

We intend our policy to be sensitive to the needs of different ethnic groups. For some young people, it is not culturally appropriate for them to be taught particular items in mixed groups. We will respond to parental requests and concerns.

Students with special needs

We will ensure that all young people receive sex and relationship education, and we will offer provision appropriate to the particular needs of all our students, taking specialist advice where necessary.

Sexual identity and sexual orientation

We aim to deal sensitively and honesty with issues of sexual orientation, answer appropriate questions and offer support. Young people, whatever their developing sexuality, need to feel that sex and relationship education is relevant to them.

8. Right to withdraw students from Sex and Relationship Education

Some parents prefer to take the responsibility for aspects of this element of education. They have the right to withdraw their children from all or part of the sex and relationship education, except for those parts included in the statutory National Curriculum (i.e. in science lessons). We would make alternative arrangements in such cases. Parents are encouraged to discuss their decisions with staff at the earliest opportunity. Parents are also welcome to review any SRE resources the group uses.

9. Confidentiality, and controversial and sensitive issues

It is advised that confidentiality is further addressed in a separate policy—one that covers more topic areas than just SRE (e.g. drug education, confidentiality for staff); however, confidentiality still needs to be commented on within the SRE policy.

Leaders cannot offer unconditional confidentiality. In a case where a leader learns from an under 16 year old that he or she is having or contemplating sexual intercourse:

- the young person will be encouraged, wherever possible, to talk to a parent/carer and if necessary seek medical advice
- child protection issues will be considered, and the young person will be referred if necessary to the leader responsible for child protection under the organisation's procedures
- the young person will be properly counselled about contraception, including precise information about where young people can access contraception and advice services.

In any case where child protection procedures are followed, the leader will ensure that the young person understands that if confidentiality has to be broken, the young person will be informed first.

Health professionals in school are bound by their codes of conduct in a one-to-one situation with an individual student, but in a group situation they must follow the organisation's confidentiality policy.

(Insert the signatures of the lead professional for the organisation/a representative from a regulatory body/a young person)

Signature..

Signature..

Young Person Representative
Signature..

Date..

Influences on sexual activity

The external influences on sexual activity are manifold, but they generally fall into three camps: family, friends and the media. For example, if a family has strong religious beliefs, there can be an expectation of no sex before marriage. On one hand this can be protective for young people, leading to delayed sexual activity and placing strong value on a relationship before sexual activity. However, it can mean that young people miss out on vital information that they may need if they find themselves in a relationship, and may feel a lot of guilt and fear for 'disobeying' parents, and/or a religious group.

Peers are another strong influence. There is a lot of talk about who's doing what with whom; and this may lead young people to experiment with sexual activity before they may have done without this influence. The irony is that most of the time it is all talk, and they are not doing what they say they are doing!

 Watch the NHS Choices video on Teen Relationships, which covers peer pressure in relation to having sex:
http://tinyurl.com/yl4hgfz

The media: TV, film, magazines and the music scene provide a stream of messages regarding sex and sexuality. These often give a good image of the glamour and excitement of sex but not the nitty-gritty concerning condom use, contraception and unplanned pregnancy.

Our role is to help young people form their own opinions regarding sex and relationships based on all the information available, and to help them form strategies to stick by their decisions. We should also help them come up with contingency plans if they find themselves in an unforeseen situation. For example, a young person may decide to be abstinent for the foreseeable future or until marriage; however, he or she needs to know how pregnancy happens, what contraception is and where to access it.

Influences on sexual activity

Divide the class into four groups titled religious groups, the media, friends and family. Give each group a piece of flip-chart paper and some markers. Have each group list what messages and values they receive from the area assigned to them regarding sex and sexuality. If the group is mixed sex, the facilitator may want to divide the class into eight groups, creating a male and female group for each topic. It could be interesting to see the different messages between the sexes.

1 Have each group present their list and encourage any additions from other participants. Tape the sheets on the wall so everyone can easily view them.

2 Have each participant come up with their own personal list of values related to sex and sexuality from the main list and add any not mentioned. Students should identify which values are uniquely theirs. Which would they never compromise on?

3 Divide a piece of paper into two columns. In the first column, invite the groups to list sayings or situations that would put them at risk of giving into peer pressure to have sex as a teen. In the second column, have the groups write what they could do to prevent the situation or how they could react to it once it happens. (For example, if you are drunk at a party, don't drink more; if you know you will be drinking, ask a friend to watch out for you.)

Sex and the media

Select some current adverts from magazines. Either individually, in small groups or as a group, ask the young people to examine the adverts. Use the sheet to direct discussion.

Sex in advertising

1 What is the product being sold by the advert?
2 Who is the target audience for this advert? (Include age range, culture, gender, race and socio-economic level.)
3 What underlying message or value is being sold by the advert? Is it obvious or subliminal?
4 Do you agree/disagree with this message?
5 Which aspect of human sexuality is being appealed to? (Emotional? Physical? Spiritual? Biological?)
6 In this a positive or negative portrayal of sexuality?

In 'couple' advertisements:
1 What is the woman doing?
2 What is the man doing?
3 Who is in the foreground?
4 Who is in the background?
5 How is juxtaposition used to convey meaning?
6 Is the woman or man placed beside objects that send out specific messages?
7 Who is active?
8 Who is not?
9 Is one person more eroticised than another?
10 What is the message you receive about this relationship?
11 Who has the power in this relationship?
12 Is this a positive or negative depiction of relationships and sexuality?

EXPLORING VALUES AND OPINIONS ABOUT RELATIONSHIPS

These activities help young people explore their values and opinions about relationships, where these values have come from, and whether they are well founded.

 Hang four signs numbered 1, 2, 3 and 4 in each corner of the room. Inform students that you will read a relationship situation. Each situation calls for a decision to be made, and you will give them four choices. They must make a decision about that situation and move to the corner of the room that indicates their choice. Remind the young people that there is no 'right answer' in each situation.

Lisa: *'I cheated on my boyfriend because the relationship had become so predictable and I needed some excitement. He never found out, and I'm not sure if I should tell him.'*

    Choice 1—Come clean and tell your boyfriend the truth.

    Choice 2—Tell him you're bored and try to improve your relationship.

    Choice 3—Do nothing; what he doesn't know can't hurt him.

    Choice 4—Break up—face it, it's over.

Amy: *'My best friend has been starting to date this much older guy; she's 15 and he's like 21. She says she likes him because he's more mature than the boys our age, he buys her stuff and he has a car. I know he's been asking her to have sex with him. I have a really bad feeling about this guy. I don't know if I should tell her what I think.'*

    Choice 1—Stay out of it; it's none of your business.

    Choice 2—You should tell her your concerns about his age; after all, she is your best friend.

    Choice 3—What this guy is doing is illegal! You should tell her parents.

    Choice 4—Go straight to the guy and ask him what he wants with your friend.

Melissa: *'My friend Nicole has been having sex with her boyfriend, and I know they aren't using contraception. She told me she's afraid to go on the pill because she doesn't want to get fat and he doesn't like condoms because they don't feel as good. They are doing the withdrawal method. I just learned in health class that withdrawal is not effective. Should I tell her she's playing with fire?'*

    Choice 1—Tell her today! She should also know she can get an STI that way.

    Choice 2—Withdrawal is better than nothing—don't say anything.

    Choice 3—So what if she gets pregnant? It would be fun to have a baby around.

    Choice 4—Tell her, and tell her you also learned that the pill doesn't make you fat. Take her to the nearest clinic.

Monique: *'My best friend has been dating this guy Jason and she thinks she is in love with him. He's such a player and I saw him kissing another girl. I'm not sure if I should tell my friend since she really likes him.'*

Choice 1—Don't tell; it's not your business.

Choice 2—Definitely tell her, she needs to know he's playing around.

Choice 3—Talk to Jason and demand that he confess to your friend.

Choice 4—Try and hint to your friend without being direct about it.

Matt: *'I just started seeing Kate, who is great. Now Chanelle, this hottie I've had a crush on all year, is totally into me. I wanna hook up with Lee this weekend, but I don't want to hurt Kate.'*

Choice 1—Hook up with Lee; you're not that serious with Kate anyway.

Choice 2—Talk to Kate about ending things.

Choice 3—Tell Lee you're interested, but taken.

Choice 4—Stay true to Kate; don't hook up with Lee.

Dwight: *'Me and my girl have been together for almost a whole year. I really love her and know she's the one for me. Her parents are really strict though, so we don't get much alone time. Recently this girl in my class who is hot for me started texting me. We started emailing all these sexual things to each other, like positions and things that turn us on, but we've never kissed or anything. Now I'm worried that my girl will find out and get really mad.'*

Choice 1—Come clean with your girlfriend; you need to be upfront with her.

Choice 2—Stop emailing this girl but don't tell your girlfriend. It will just upset her.

Choice 3—If your girlfriend won't find out, what's the harm of a little email?

Choice 4—Your girlfriend's not giving you what you need; you should tell her you need more or else you're going to move on.

ARE YOU IN A GOOD RELATIONSHIP?

The following is a light-hearted activity, but it introduces the concept of a relationship being something that builds each partner up and helps each one to grow, where each member can be unguarded and open, and doesn't break down self-worth.

How good is your relationship?

The following quiz can be used to evaluate any type of relationship, including a romantic relationship, friendship or family relationship.

After the students have had time to complete the worksheet, ask them to score their answers by giving one point for a 'yes' response to questions 2, 3, 4, 6, 9, 11, 12, 13 and 14. Also give one point for each 'no' response to questions 1, 5, 7, 8 and 10.

Scores:

1–3: There are few constructive elements in this relationship. You may want to think about your reasons for continuing the relationship, or work toward improving it.

4–6: This relationship has problems that might be resolved by working on honesty and communication.

7–10: There is the basis for a good relationship. . Focus on the positive elements and work on improving the destructive ones.

10–14: You're doing well and have what it takes to build a successful and satisfying relationship.

Adapted from: Hubbard. *Entering Adulthood: Living in Relationships*. Network Publications; 1990.

Evaluating a relationship

Answer each question by circling yes or no.

1	Do you feel that the other person in this relationship does not understand you?	**YES / NO**
2	Are you able to speak freely to him or her about things that bother you?	**YES / NO**
3	Do you take a genuine interest in each other's lives?	**YES / NO**
4	Do both of you pursue individual interests?	**YES / NO**
5	Is this relationship the only important relationship in your life?	**YES / NO**
6	Do you believe that you are a worthwhile person outside of this relationship?	**YES / NO**
7	Do you expect this person to meet all of your emotional or physical needs?	**YES / NO**
8	Is your relationship often threatened by others?	**YES / NO**
9	Can you be yourself in this relationship?	**YES / NO**
10	Are you uncomfortable sharing your feelings with this person?	**YES / NO**
11	Do you both work to improve the relationship?	**YES / NO**
12	Do you feel good about yourself?	**YES / NO**
13	Do you feel you have become a better person because of this relationship?	**YES / NO**
14	Can you both accept changes in roles and feelings within the relationship?	**YES / NO**

CHAPTER 9

Contraception and young people

Teenagers use of and access to contraception continues to raise heated debate. There are those who feel all contraceptive methods should be easily available to all ages, including those who are legally under the age of consent, and those who feel that increasing availability encourages sexual activity and risk taking.

What is certain is that myths surrounding contraception still abound in all ages. This is despite vast improvements in recent years to the quality and consistency of sexual health information provided, e.g. the PSHE curriculum including standard information on all contraceptive methods.

A survey for Doctor magazine highlighted a worrying lack of understanding about contraception among UK teenagers. One teenager was quoted as saying: 'Putting a watch around your penis before sex means the radioactivity of the dial kills off sperm.' Others believed a Coca-Cola douche, standing on a telephone directory, or drinking a lot of milk would stop them getting pregnant. Still others thought they could not get pregnant if they stayed upside down for two hours, coughed immediately after sex, or had sex in the bath, on a boat, or with their clothes on.

About 8 000 teenagers under 16 get pregnant every year in the UK, and rates of sexually transmitted infection in British teenagers are running at about 10%. Contraception use is neither universal nor consistent. It is worth noting here that teenagers requesting pregnancy termination are no less responsible about contraceptive use at the time of conception than older women.[1] Older teenagers are actually the main age group attending contraception services. This figure dramatically reduces for those 15 and under.

NHS Contraceptive Services, England: 2007–08

- The peak age group for clinic attendance was 16–19, based on the rate per 100 population; an estimated 20% of women in this age group visited a clinic during the year. The equivalent figure for 15 year olds and under is 8%.
- Oral contraception remains the most popular form of contraception among women, accounting for 46% of female contraceptive use.
- Use of Long-Acting Reversible Contraceptives (LARCs) continues to increase and now accounts for 23% of primary methods of contraception, compared to 21% the previous year and 18% in 2003–04. LARCs include: intrauterine device (IUD), injectable contraception, implants and intrauterine system (IUS).
- Emergency hormonal contraception (EHC) became available over the counter (OTC) in pharmacies in 2001–02. Consequently, emergency contraception issued by clinics has fallen by 30%, compared to 2001–02, and was issued on about 136 000 occasions in 2006–07, a fall of 22 000 (14%) on the previous year.

Source: www.ic.nhs.uk/pubs/nhscontra0708 (Accessed 28 October 2008).

The most significant change in the contraception field over the past decade has been the increasing availability of LARC to all age groups and particularly young people. Inserting the contraceptive implant and intrauterine devices have become wider practiced skills, and the myth that women who have not had children cannot have an IUD inserted is being dispelled. In fact, the IUD is increasingly being fitted as a form of emergency contraception.

The National Institute of Clinical Excellence (NICE) clinical guideline on LARC offers the best-practice advice for all women of reproductive age who may wish to regulate their fertility by using LARC methods.

Additional resources

Long-Acting Reversible Contraception: quick reference guide. **NICE** (2005). Available at: www.nice.org.uk

In addition, the emergency pill has become more widely available, most notably through becoming an over-the-counter medication that can be accessed directly from pharmacies. Many areas have schemes to make this cost free for those aged 18 or under.

Find out from your community health service pharmacist which local pharmacies are involved in this scheme. Leaflets can be made available to the young people using your service. Arrange a visit to the local pharmacist for a small group of young people to raise awareness of what a pharmacy can provide.

This chapter aims to equip professionals to answer young people's questions regarding contraception and to facilitate a session about contraception. It covers basic information on contraceptive methods and contraceptive myths and suggests activities to explore beliefs and practice around contraception. This information would be supported by information in Chapter 1: Puberty and periods.

STOP PRESS!

A sexually active teenager who does not use contraception has a 90% chance of conceiving within a year. Yet contraception isn't always high on the agenda when teens become sexually active. Various pregnancy myths such as 'it's OK on my period' or 'not on the first time' persist. Young people worry over confidentiality, knowing where to access contraception and whether it is legal to use contraception. This stops young people asking for contraceptive advice. Young people are afraid of the effect hormonal contraception may have, they don't always understand how to use the method, and their partner doesn't always support them in seeking or using contraception.

Not using contraception properly accounts for the majority of unintended pregnancies in contraceptive users. Teenagers are generally poor contraception users and delay seeking advice until crisis management is required. Even when they are using a contraceptive method, the failure rates are higher for adolescents than older women.

Once the method relies on the user for efficacy, the failure rates increase. With the lowest failure rates, implants and injections are the most effective methods of contraception for young people. This is probably as they do not rely on the user remembering to take tablets, change a patch, or to use a condom when having sex.

SO WHAT ABOUT ABSTINENCE?

Abstaining from sex is a failsafe way of avoiding the risk of pregnancy or sexually transmitted infections (STIs). Delaying sex, sticking with one partner and using contraception (and particularly condoms) are the next-best option for avoiding pregnancy and STIs.

Abstinence should always be discussed in a session about contraception; research has shown that when young people delay sexual activity they have fewer partners, are less likely to acquire STIs and are less likely to regret sexual intercourse. Conversely, there is no point in promoting abstinence only without discussion of contraception and STI prevention, as although abstinence may be an ideal, if a young person does embark on a sexual relationship he or she can make informed decisions regarding starting a family and protecting him or herself from infection. Abstinence-only programmes have been shown to be ineffective in America, which has high rates of teenage pregnancy.

 Discuss with your group the pros and cons of abstinence. Get the group to think about what some of the reasons might be for a young person to choose to be abstinent. What are the qualities a person might need to remain abstinent within a relationship? What might make a person's wish to be abstinent fail?

Some reasons young people choose to be abstinent or to postpone sex

Personal:
- personal values or religious/moral beliefs
- not ready yet
- to avoid guilt, fear or disappointment.

Medical:
- to avoid pregnancy
- to avoid STIs
- health and protection against disease, e.g. the risk factors for cervical can-cer include: early age of first intercourse, higher number of sexual part-ners, and younger age at first pregnancy.

Relational:
- haven't met the right person
- to strengthen a relationship. Abstaining or postponing sexual activity may allow time to develop a deeper friendship and establish intimacy that is not sexual.

What are some qualities that will help maintain abstinence or postpone sexual activity?

- Ability to resist pressure.
- Respect for the other person's feelings.
- High degree of self-control.

What are some reasons that a commitment to be abstinent or postpone sexual activity might fail?

- Fear of saying no.
- Pressure from your partner.
- Peer pressure—'everyone is doing it'.
- Wanting to be loved.
- Use of alcohol or drugs.

A ROUGH GUIDE TO CONTRACEPTION

The following is a rough guide to contraception. The fact sheets can be printed and used as handouts. Before starting a session on contraception it is always a good idea to ask the class what contraception is. Acknowledge that people may have different beliefs or ideas about this, but that the purpose of the session is to give information so that people can make informed choices if they become sexually active.

 It can be helpful for some young people to be able to ask questions about sex and contraception anonymously. If the session is announced in advance, a sealed box can be made available where they can post their questions.

Where can you get contraception?

Hormonal and intrauterine contraception is available through dedicated community contraception and sexual health clinics, as well as Departments of Sexual Health within hospitals (sometimes called genito-urinary medicine services, or GUM), and general practice surgeries.

Emergency contraception is available through additional sources such as A&E departments, the school nurse and over the counter at pharmacies.

Condoms are available from contraception and sexual health clinics, various commercial outlets (usually pharmacies), some bars and nightclubs, some GPs and various community schemes.

Check out the NHS Choices website for mini videos that could be used to spark debate with your group around contraception: www.nhs.uk/video

Types of contraception: http://tinyurl.com/yhest3x

Where to get contraception: http://tinyurl.com/y9gq9he

Condom negotiation: http://tinyurl.com/y9z7n6s

Teenagers and contraception: http://tinyurl.com/y9anmo3

MALE CONDOM

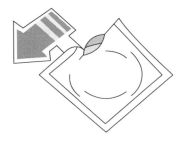

Efficacy:

The male condom is 98% effective.

How does it work?

It is put over an erect penis to catch sperm and prevent it entering the vagina.

Advantages:

- as well as stopping pregnancy, condoms are the only method that also protect against STIs (this includes the female condom)
- condoms come in different varieties. They can be different flavours, colours, ribbed, be made of latex or polyurethane and be sensitive or extra strong.

Disadvantages:

- condom use must be negotiated between both partners
- may be seen as interrupting sex.

Possible problems:

- burst, split or slipped condom during sexual intercourse
- allergy to the condom
- loss of sensation.

HOW TO PUT ON A CONDOM

Step 1	Check for CE mark—the European standard mark (indication of quality standard, that the condom has been tested). Check that the condom is in date. Check for tears and rips in the packet. Any hole in the packet will mean the condom has dried out and may split. It is best to keep condoms in a dry, cool place. Put the condom on when the penis is erect, before there is any contact between the penis and your partner's body. Fluid released from the penis during the early stages of an erection (pre-ejaculate) can contain sperm.
Step 2	Push the condom down to the bottom of the packet and carefully tear the top. Teeth and nails can make a hole in the condom. Tear along one side of the foil, being sure not to rip the condom inside. Carefully remove the condom.
Step 3	Air trapped inside a condom could cause it to break. To avoid this, squeeze the closed end of the condom between your forefinger and thumb and place the condom over the erect penis. Be sure that the roll is on the outside. If you find the condom is on upside down and isn't rolling, throw it away and start again. If you just turn it around there will be sperm on the outside from the pre-ejaculate.
Step 4	While still squeezing the closed end, use your other hand to unroll the condom gently down the full length of the penis.
Step 5	Soon after ejaculation, withdraw the penis while it is still erect by holding the condom firmly in place. Remove the condom only when the penis is fully withdrawn. Keep both the penis and condom clear from contact with your partner's body.
Step 6	Dispose of the used condom hygienically. Wrap the condom in a tissue and place it in a bin (do not flush it down the toilet).

Figure 9.1 How to use a condom

The following list is a compilation of common 'excuses' that people use to avoid using condoms. Each 'excuse' is presented with a possible response to help better negotiate condom use and improve communication on these issues. This could be used as a handout to support discussion around condom use.

Condom Excuses

'I can't feel anything when I wear a condom.'

'I know there's a little less sensation, but there's not a lot less. Why don't we put a drop of lubricant inside the condom? That'll make it feel more sensitive.'

'If I have to stop and put it on, I won't be in the mood anymore.'

'I can help you put it on. That way, you'll continue to be aroused, and we'll both be protected.'

'I don't need to use a condom. I haven't had sex in ___ months, so I know I don't have any diseases.'

'That's good to know. As far as I know, I'm disease-free, too. But I'd still like to use a condom because either of us could have an infection and not know it.'

'Condoms are messy, and they smell funny.

It's really not that bad. And sex can be a little messy sometimes. But this way, we'll be able to enjoy it and both be protected from pregnancy and STIs.'

'Let's not use condoms just this once.'

'No. Once is all it takes to get pregnant or get an infection.'

'I don't have a condom with me.'

'That's okay. I do.'

'You never asked me to use a condom before. Are you having an affair?'

'No. I just think we made a mistake by never using condoms before. One of us could have an infection and not know it. It's best to be safe.'

'If you really loved me, you wouldn't make me wear one.'

'If you really loved me, you'd want to protect yourself—and me—from infections and pregnancy so that we can be together and healthy for a long time.'

'Why are you asking me to wear a condom? Do you think I'm dirty or something?'

'It's not about being dirty or clean. It's about avoiding pregnancy and the risk of infection.'

'Only people who have anal sex need to wear condoms, and I'm not like that.'

'That's not true. A person can get an infection during any kind of sex, including what we do together.'

'Condoms don't fit me.'

'Condoms can stretch a lot—in fact, they can stretch to fit over a person's head! So we should be able to find one that fits you.'

'Why should we use condoms? They just break.'

'Actually, they told me that condoms are tested before they're sent out—so while they have been known to break, it happens rarely, especially if you know how to use one correctly—and I do.'

'If you don't want to get pregnant, why don't you just take the birth control pill?'

'Because the birth control pill only protects against pregnancy. The condom protects against both pregnancy and infections.'

FEMALE CONDOM 'FEMIDOM'

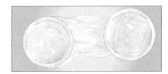

Efficacy

The female condom is 95% effective.

How does it work?

The Femidom is a pre-lubricated, soft, polyurethane sheath that lines the vagina and acts as a barrier to sperm entering the vagina. There is a smaller inner ring and larger outer ring. The smaller inner ring is used to feed the femidom into the vagina. Most of the femidom goes inside the woman and the larger ring overlaps the outer area of the vagina.

Advantages:

- the woman has control over use
- it protects against STIs.

Disadvantages:

- some people find them noisy
- it may be seen as interrupting sex.

Possible problems:

- penis inserted outside the female condom
- noise—some women have commented about a rustling noise.

How to use a femidom

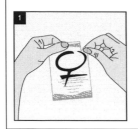	Open the package carefully; tear at the notch on the top right of the package. Do not use scissors or a knife to open.
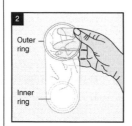	The outer ring covers the area around the opening of the vagina. The inner ring is used for insertion and to help hold the sheath in place during intercourse.
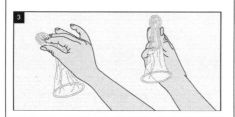	While holding the sheath at the closed end, grasp the flexible inner ring and squeeze it with the thumb and second or middle finger so it becomes long and narrow.
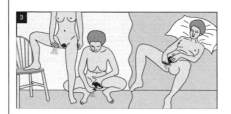	Choose a position that is comfortable for insertion—squat, raise one leg, sit or lie down.
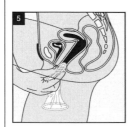	Gently insert the inner ring into the vagina. Feel the inner ring go up and move into place.
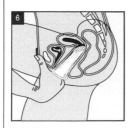	Place the index finger on the inside of the condom, and push the inner ring up as far as it will go. Be sure the sheath is not twisted. The outer ring should remain on the outside of the vagina.

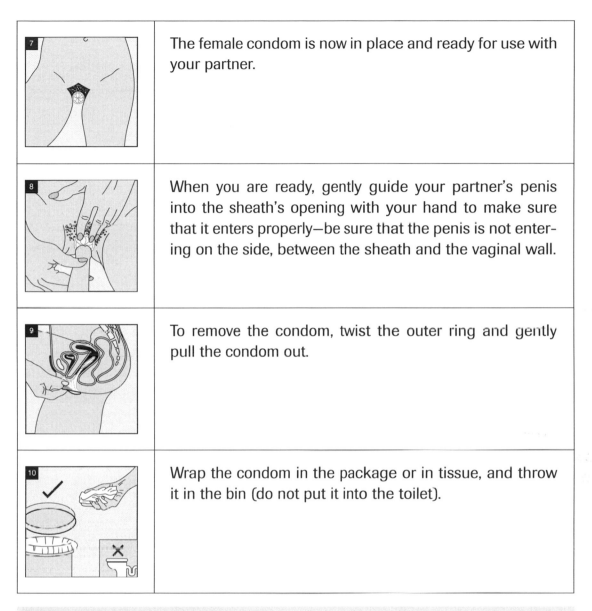

	The female condom is now in place and ready for use with your partner.
	When you are ready, gently guide your partner's penis into the sheath's opening with your hand to make sure that it enters properly—be sure that the penis is not entering on the side, between the sheath and the vaginal wall.
	To remove the condom, twist the outer ring and gently pull the condom out.
	Wrap the condom in the package or in tissue, and throw it in the bin (do not put it into the toilet).

Figure 9.2 How to use a femidom

Ideally the 'Double Dutch' method should be recommended. This is where the young woman uses a reliable form of hormonal contraception as well as condoms, just in case the condom splits or comes off.

THE COMBINED PILL

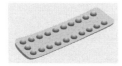

Efficacy

The combined pill is over 99% effective if taken according to instructions.

How does it work?

The combined pill contains hormones that copy our natural hormones (oestrogen and progestogen). The pills stop ovulation whilst they are being taken. It also makes cervical mucus thicker, which stops sperm getting to an egg. Pills are taken for three weeks, then there is a week's break. During the break there will probably be a short, light bleed. This is not a real period, but what is called a withdrawal bleed caused by the level of hormones dropping whilst the pill is not being taken.

Advantages:

• the user is in control of the method
• there is a quick return of fertility after stopping use
• it often makes bleeds lighter and less painful
• the combined pill is protective against womb and ovarian cancer.

Disadvantages:

• the user is in control of the method; it needs to be taken regularly to be effective
• rare side effects may include deep vein thrombosis (DVT), breast cancer and cervical cancer.

Possible side effects:

• nausea (often short-term)
• breast tenderness and swelling (often short-term)
• breakthrough bleeding
• depression
• changes in libido
• application site reactions.

THE PATCH

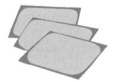

Efficacy

The contraceptive patch is 99% effective.

How does it work?

The patches contain oestrogen and progestogen. The hormones are absorbed through the skin, stop ovulation and thicken cervical mucus. The patch can be put on your arm, thigh, back shoulder or buttock. One patch is worn each week for three weeks and then there is a patch-free week.

Advantages:

- some side effects may be less than with the combined pill as the hormones are released straight into the bloodstream rather than having to go through the liver first
- only three patch changes per cycle
- the user is in control of method
- there is a quick return of fertility after stopping use
- it often makes bleeds lighter and less painful
- as it is similar to the combined pill, the patch may be protective against womb and ovarian cancer
- daily activities such as bathing, showering, swimming and exercise can all be continued as normal without the patch coming off.

Disadvantages:

- the user is in control of the method, and the patch needs to be changed at weekly intervals to be effective
- as the hormones are similar to the combined pill, side effects such as DVT and cancers are the same
- the patch is visible.

Possible side effects:

- nausea
- breast tenderness
- break through bleeding
- depression
- changes in libido
- Application site reactions.

THE PROGESTOGEN-ONLY PILL

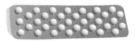

Efficacy

The progestogen-only pill is 99% effective if taken according to instructions.

How does it work?

The hormone progestogen thickens cervical mucus to stop sperm meeting an egg. In some women, it stops ovulation. This pill is taken every day without a break.

Advantages:

- the client is in control of method
- there is a quick return in fertility
- it can be used whilst breastfeeding
- it is suitable for women who are unable to use the combined pill.

Disadvantages:

- it needs to be taken carefully
- periods may be irregular.

Possible side effects:

- ovarian cysts
- breast tenderness
- feeling bloated
- depression
- variations in weight
- nausea
- irregular/no bleeding.

INJECTION

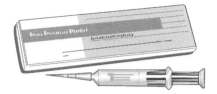

Efficacy

The Depo-Provera injection is over 99% effective.

How does it work?

An injection is given, usually in your bum (although it can be given in the arm or thigh), once every three months. It is just one hormone, progestogen, and stops ovulation whilst the hormone is in the system.

Advantages:

* only one injection every 12 weeks
* the user is not involved
* this method usually stops periods as it keeps the womb lining at the same thickness, and there is no build up of blood

Disadvantages:

* user may have some irregular bleeding or spotting initially
* once given, it cannot be withdrawn
* after stopping the injection, it can take up to a year for ovulation to reoccur, but for some fertility comes back as soon as an injection is due.

Possible side effects:

* headaches
* feeling bloated
* depression
* weight gain
* mood swings
* irregular/no bleeding.

IUD (INTRAUTERINE DEVICE)

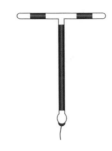

Efficacy

The IUD is 98% to over 99% effective.

How does it work?

The IUD is a small plastic device shaped like a T, with thin copper wire wrapped around it. It sits in your womb and is fitted by a doctor or nurse. The copper is noxious to sperm and eggs and stops them meeting. The IUD lasts for up to 10 years, although you can have it taken out whenever you want.

Advantages:

- it works immediately
- there are no hormones involved
- it is immediately reversible
- the user is not involved.

Disadvantages:

- can make periods heavier and longer.
- needs to be inserted and removed by a doctor or nurse.

Possible side effects:

- heavier, more painful periods
- increased risk of ectopic pregnancy if the IUD fails (minimal)
- increased risk of pelvic infection
- malposition or expulsion of IUD
- pregnancy due to malposition or expulsion of IUD.

INTRAUTERINE SYSTEM (IUS), OR 'MIRENA'

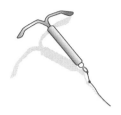

Efficacy:
The IUS is over 99% effective.

How does it work?
The IUS is a small plastic device with a slow-releasing hormone in the stem. It sits in your womb and is inserted and removed by a doctor or nurse. The hormone in it is progestogen and it works by thickening the cervical mucus to stop sperm meeting an egg. It also makes the womb lining unfavourable to implantation. The IUS works for up to five years. As it works in a different way to the IUD, the Mirena is not effective as emergency contraception.

Advantages:
- the user is not involved
- periods will be much lighter, shorter and less painful
- periods may stop.

Disadvantages:
- there may be some irregular bleeding
- it needs to be inserted and removed by a doctor or nurse
- there is a risk of expulsion or malposition
- pregnancy due to expulsion or malposition of IUS.

Possible side effects:
- breast tenderness
- acne
- headaches
- feeling bloated
- mood changes
- nausea
- irregular/no bleeding.

IMPLANT

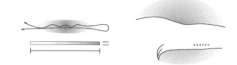

Efficacy:

The implant is over 99% effective.

How does it work?

It is a small, soft tube the size of a matchstick, inserted by a doctor or nurse under the skin of the upper arm. It is not visible but can be felt under the skin. Like the injection, it releases a small amount of progestogen every day and stops ovulation. It also makes the cervical mucous thicker and presents a barrier to sperm getting through. It lasts for three years.

Advantages:

- it works immediately
- the user is not involved.
- lasts 3 years.

Disadvantages:

- bleeding pattern can be unpredictable
- requires insertion and removal by a doctor or nurse.

Possible side effects:

- irregular or no bleeding
- nausea
- vomiting
- headache
- dizziness
- breast discomfort
- depression
- skin disorders
- disturbance of appetite/weight changes
- changes in libido.

THE EMERGENCY PILL

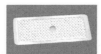

Efficacy

The emergency pill (Levonelle) is more effective the sooner it is taken. It can be taken up to three days (72 hours) after unprotected sexual intercourse. There is a new emergency pill available; its efficacy stays the same for 5 days ('Ella One').

How does it work?

The emergency pill is made from the hormone progestogen. Depending on where in the woman's cycle it is taken, it either delays ovulation so there is no egg for the sperm to reach, or if there is a fertilised egg, stops it from implanting.

Advantages:

- effective at preventing pregnancy
- the woman is in control of the method
- it can be used after unprotected sexual intercourse.

Disadvantages:

- it doesn't provide future contraception
- it may disrupt the next period
- it is less effective the later it is taken (Levonelle)
- it cannot be used if there is a risk of pregnancy previously in the cycle (Ella One).

Possible side effects:

- nausea and vomiting
- breast tenderness
- headache
- dizziness
- fatigue
- bleeding patterns may be temporarily disturbed.

Contraceptive values

This activity allows the young people to explore his or her own thoughts around becoming sexually active and the use or non-use of contraception.

Place headings around the room indicating a range of acceptance levels for different statements. Headings include:

- yes, strongly agree
- yes, agree
- neutral
- no, disagree
- no, strongly disagree.

Ask the young people to stand under or near the sign that best describes their values or beliefs in response to each of the following statements, one statement at a time. Remind the young people that everyone has a right to his or her own opinion. Ensure confidentiality is reinforced.

Statements:

- it is mainly the guy's responsibility to buy condoms
- teens who abstain from sex are less likely to be harmed emotionally
- teens who abstain from sex are less likely to be harmed physically
- if you can't talk with your partner about sex or contraception ahead of time, then you shouldn't even consider having sex
- i would not buy condoms from a shop where I might know someone
- Having sex without using contraception for the first one or two times is OK because the chances of getting pregnant are minimal.

After each statement is read and the young people have placed themselves beneath a heading, encourage the students to explain why they choose to stand under one heading over another. Use the following questions to guide the discussion:

- what made you decide to stand where you did?
- how does your decision to stand there affect other people?
- are you comfortable where you are standing?
- would there be a situation that would make you stand somewhere different?

True/false game

This game has a similar format but is more lighthearted.

Place large cards with the words 'true' and 'false' at each end of the room. Read out a statement from the following myths and truths sheets (or think of some of your own) and ask the young people to put themselves on either 'true' or 'false' (or stay in the middle if they don't know the answer). This will raise discussion, as well as cause great hilarity; naturally, make sure the facts are emphasized.

A lot of these myths will come up if you have a discussion about contraceptive methods before using the fact sheets.

Myths and truths

You can't get pregnant the first time you have sex—false!

- Some people believe an intact hymen (the thin skin that stretches across part of the opening of the vagina) can stop you becoming pregnant the first time you have sex. But it doesn't cover the cervix, and you can become pregnant any time you have sex unless you use contraception to protect yourself.

You can get pregnant even if you have sex standing up—true!

- You can become pregnant by having sex in any position unless you use quality reliable contraception to protect yourself.

You can get pregnant just from kissing or touching—false!

- You can't become pregnant just from kissing or touching your partner unless you allow sperm to come in contact with the vagina. It is important to remember any contact between your vagina and your partner's sperm could result in a pregnancy.

I can still get pregnant even if I wash after sex—true!

- Some people believe washing their vagina after sex will somehow kill or wash out the sperm. In fact, what it actually does is push the sperm up higher into the vagina, so it has an even better chance of finding the egg. You also risk the chance of irritation if using anything other than water to wash.

I can get pregnant if I've never had my period—true!

- Remember, your period comes at the end of your fertility cycle. It happens because there are no egg and sperm meeting, so the blood lining the uterus is being discarded. Many girls have become pregnant because they had sex during their first egg cycle.

I can't get pregnant if he pulls out in time—false!

- Even pre-ejaculatory fluid contains millions of sperm, making it possible for you to become pregnant even if your partner doesn't ejaculate inside you.

I can still get pregnant while I have my period—true!

- You can become pregnant at any time during your monthly cycle. Even though it's possible to predict when a woman is least fertile, there is no guaranteed safe time. Remember, sperm can live in a woman's body for up to seven days waiting for an egg to be released.

You can't get pregnant the first time—false!
- If you have started your periods, you are releasing eggs. If there are eggs and sperm about, they could meet and you could become pregnant—even the first time you have sex.

'X' contraceptive method will stop me from having children when I am older—false!
- All methods of hormonal contraception are reversible. There are no long-term effects on a woman's fertility if she has used a hormonal method of contraception.

The pill makes you put on weight—false!
- Recent studies have shown that this is not the case and the weight gain that you observe when someone is taking the pill for months to years would have been a natural weight gain anyway!

You can't have a coil fitted if you haven't had children—false!
- Any woman can have an IUD fitted, even if she hasn't had children. In fact, the IUD is often fitted as a form of emergency contraception if a woman presents late for the emergency pill but up to five days after unprotected sex.
- Some health professionals are concerned regarding a young woman's risk of infection if she is not with a regular partner. Also, if you've had a vaginal delivery, your cervix will have been stretched by the baby coming through it and it is easier to fit an IUD—so some health professionals prefer to only fit an IUD if you've already had a child. However, it is possible to fit an IUD for someone who hasn't had children, and if you need an emergency IUD fitted or it is your chosen method, you should be directed to an organisation that will do this for you.

You can only take the emergency pill one or two times—false!
- It is safe to take the emergency pill as many times as needed; there will be no bad effects on your body or fertility. What it can do is interrupt your periods, so if you have to take it many times close together it is very difficult to know when your eggs are going to be around, and therefore unprotected sex is very risky. Also, it is not 100% effective, so it would be far better to use a reliable ongoing method of contraception to avoid the uncertainty and inconvenience of having to use the emergency pill lots of times.

In a group, look at the following news item. Encourage debate about the issues raised, language use, accuracy of information given, and effect of the media on popular opinion.

Teenagers offered implants to stop pregnancy

Teenage girls will be steered towards long-term contraceptives in the battle to reduce the number of underage pregnancies. Many fail to take the traditional pill regularly and cannot use condoms properly. These methods are having little impact on the teenage pregnancy rate, which remains the highest in western Europe. The alternatives—such as contraceptive injections and implants, and intrauterine devices (coils)—do not need to be topped up every day and last between three months and five years.

The policy, backed with a £26.8million cash injection to the Health Service, could lead to a dramatic fall in the estimated 400 000 unwanted pregnancies each year. But family rights campaigners warned that the move would encourage promiscuity and could fuel the rise in sexually-transmitted infections such as chlamydia. Others expressed fears about side effects associated with the long-acting reversible contraceptives (LARCs).

Although Britain's rate of teenage pregnancies has fallen from the peak years of the late 1990s, it is still the second highest in the Western world after the U.S. The Department of Health said it wants to see greater use of LARCs because the success of condoms and contraceptive pills depends on "correct and consistent use".

At the moment, only 14 per cent of women use LARCs. But family planning clinics will be encouraged to use them rather than simply dishing out condoms and the Pill. £14million is earmarked for "innovative new ways" of helping young people get access to sexual health advice and contraception.

Discussion points

1   Is contraception use or non-use the main reason for high rates of teenage pregnancy? (Consider other factors such as family values, religious beliefs and practices, aspirations, role models, etc.)

2   In the light of this, do you think the government claim that long-acting reversible contraception (LARC) will lead to a dramatic fall in teenage pregnancy is well founded?

3   Does making contraception more widely available lead to increased sexual activity? (There is much evidence that says this is not the case, and in fact, knowledge around relationships, contraception and STIs has been shown to lead to delayed sexual activity.)

4   In your opinion, will there be an increased rate of STIs as contraception becomes more widely available? Why? *Research has shown that STI rates are increasing, despite pregnancy rates decreasing. This would suggest that the condom is being abandoned as other forms of contraception are becoming more accessible. We need to encourage doubling up and seeing the LARC methods or the pill as the back-up method.*

5   What do you think of the use of the word 'promiscuity' in this article?

6   What do you know about confidentiality and consent to all contraception methods for young people (including those under the age of 16)?

    If a young person is Fraser competent (*see* Chapter 7 for further details) he or she can receive contraception advice and provision without the consent or knowledge of their parents.

7   The government is encouraging innovative ways to deliver LARC to young people in addition to the traditional route of General Practice and contraception clinics. Any suggestions?

Additional resources from www.fpa.org.uk

4 Girls: a below-the-bra guide to the female body
A6 booklet
Covers: Sexual development, feelings, weight, diet, body hair, breasts, genitals, menstrual cycle, sexual health, contraception, STIs, what to do if you think you might be pregnant.

Is everybody doing it? Your guide to contraception
A6 booklet
Covers: Are you ready to have sex? Where to get information and help about contraception, brief information on STIs, condom use, how to use a condom, contraceptive methods, what to do if you think you might be pregnant.

Periods: What you need to know
A6 booklet
Covers: Reproductive system, periods, FAQ re: periods, sanitary towels and tampons, activities when on your period.

4 Boys: A below the belt guide to the male body
A6 booklet
Covers: Body changes, the male reproductive system, self-examination, masturbation, ejaculation, condoms.

Information about contraception for young people

A booklet on practical advice for young people about pregnancy and contraception called **Condoms, pills and other useful things: A young person's guide to contraception and STIs** can be **downloaded from <u>www.avert.org</u>**

Check it out

Handbook of contraception and family planning by Suzanne Everett and printed in 2000 by Balliere-Tindall.

Additional resources

Avert is an international HIV and Aids charity. The website includes details of contraceptive methods and has some good interactive quizzes on condom use and pregnancy. These quizzes can be printed.
www.avert.org

Brook offers free and confidential sexual health advice and contraception to young people up to the age of 25. The website includes simple yet detailed summaries of contraceptive methods.
www.brook.org.uk

REFERENCE

1. Harvey N, Gaudoin M. Teenagers requesting pregnancy termination are no less responsible about contraceptive use at the time of conception than older women. *BJOG.* 2007; **114**(2); 226–229.

CHAPTER 10

Sexual health

Recent figures from the Health Protection Agency show that young people have the greatest amount of sexually transmitted infection. This could be for two reasons: increased unsafe sexual behaviour and increased testing and acceptability of testing. Services are accepting that young people can be sexually active and are providing advice, guidance, infection screening and contraception.

The consequences of STIs are manifold. There is often immediate discomfort and embarrassment for the person with the STI, having one STI can facilitate the transmission of another, and having an STI can cause chronic conditions such as pain and infertility.

It is in an individual's interests to avoid getting STIs so they do not suffer the longer-term consequences; however, it is also in society's interests to prevent STI transmission as society ultimately bears the cost of treating infertility and chronic pain.

Statistics

- Young people (aged 16 to 24 years old) are the age group most at risk of being diagnosed with a sexually transmitted infection, accounting for 65% of all chlamydia, 50% of genital warts and 50% of gonorrhoea infections diagnosed in genitourinary medicine clinics across the UK in 2007.
- The most common sexually transmitted infection in young people is genital chlamydia. The National Chlamydia Screening Programme in England performed 270 729 screens in under-25 year olds in 2007: 9.5% of screens in women and 8.4% in men were positive for chlamydia. A further 79 557 diagnoses of genital chlamydia infection were made among young people in genitourinary medicine clinics in the UK in 2007, (a rate of 1 102 per 100 000 16 to 24 year olds), a rise of 7% on 2006.

- Genital warts were the second most commonly diagnosed sexually transmitted infection among young people in genitourinary medicine clinics,
  with 49 250 cases diagnosed in 2007 (682 per 100 000), a 8% rise on 2006.
- In 2007, 702 young people were diagnosed with HIV, representing 11% of
  all new HIV diagnoses. Young men who have sex with men remain the
  group of young people most at risk of acquiring HIV in the UK.

Source: Health Protection Agency. *Sexually transmitted Infections and Young
People in the United Kingdom* [report]. 2008. Available at: www.hpa.org.uk/
Publications/InfectiousDiseases/HIVAndSTIs/0807STIsyoungpeopleinUK2008

THE SEXUAL HEALTH AND HIV STRATEGY

The Sexual Health and HIV Strategy was published in 2002. The Strategy indicates
the long-term commitment to modernise and improve sexual health services.
This has been followed up with an Effective Sexual Health Promotion Toolkit.
It represents a wide range of interests and views within sexual health and health
promotion and HIV prevention and has a series of useful fact sheets for different
client groups.

Sexual Health and HIV Strategy

www.dh.gov.uk/en/Publichealth/Healthimprovement/
Sexualhealth/Sexualhealthgeneralinformation/DH_4002168

THE NATIONAL CHLAMYDIA SCREENING PROGRAMME

The National Chlamydia Screening Programme aims to test all young people 25
and under, and many agencies are involved in implementing this. Historically,
testing has been offered in health settings such as GP practices; however, increasingly innovative locations are being sought to reach those who are not keen on
visiting a health establishment. These locations include schools, colleges, roving
buses, clubs, youth group meeting places and more.

If you feel your organisation would like to offer this service, get in touch
with your local Chlamydia Screening Office—you could call the National Sexual
Health Helpline and they will be able to advise you.

Sexual Health Helpline—0800 567 123

To find out more about the National Chlamydia Screening Programme, see the following website:
www.chlamydiascreening.nhs.uk

THE INFECTIONS

There are many STIs. However, we will talk here about the most common ones. There are many good websites that have more comprehensive information:

Additional resources

Brook

Brook Advisory Centres—commonly known just as Brook—is the only national voluntary sector provider of free and confidential sexual health advice and services specifically for young people under 25.
www.brook.org.uk/content/M2_4_sti.asp

Sexually Transmitted Infections (STIs)
Straightforward but brief outline of sexually transmitted infections and their treatments. Part of the NHS Direct website.
www.nhsdirect.nhs.uk

The following fact sheets can be used in an outreach session with young people or simply for your own information. It is very important to give young people accurate and factual information around their health; there are many myths regarding how STIs are transmitted and their consequences, and it is essential that young people seek prompt advice after unprotected sex.

What causes STIs?

Bacteria

These infections and their symptoms can be cleared with treatment.

Protozoa

These infections and their symptoms can be cleared with treatment.

Fungi

These infections are not sexually transmitted but are often aggravated by sexual behaviour. The symptoms can be cleared by treatment.

Viruses

These infections cannot be cleared with treatment, *but* the symptoms can be.

Mites and lice

These infections and their symptoms can be completely cleared by treatment.

Based on an idea by, and with thanks to, Geoff Huckle, Chlamydia Screening Office, City and Hackney Community Health Services.

Chlamydia

Signs and symptoms

The majority of women who are infected with chlamydia will have no symptoms, but some may notice:

- increased vaginal discharge
- frequent or painful urination
- lower abdominal pain
- pain during sex
- irregular periods.

Men are more likely to notice symptoms, but some may not have symptoms. They may experience:

- discharge from the penis
- pain/burning on urination.

Sometimes the eyes can become infected with chlamydia and both men and women may experience painful eye swelling and irritation.

Chlamydia is a type of bacteria.

Transmission

Chlamydia can be transmitted in the following ways:

- penetrative sex (where the penis enters the vagina, mouth or anus)
- mother to baby during birth
- occasionally by transferring the infection on fingers from the genitals to the eyes.

Diagnosis and treatment

Self-samples can be done to pick up chlamydia either via a vaginal swab or urine test. The results are usually available within a week. If the test is positive, the treatment for chlamydia is a simple course of antibiotics.

Long-term effects

If left untreated, chlamydia can lead to pelvic inflammatory disease in women. This can cause fever, pain, and can lead to infertility or ectopic pregnancy.

A woman can pass it on to her baby if she is infected when the baby is born.

In men, chlamydia can cause inflammation of the testicles and the prostate gland, which causes pain. Without treatment the urethra may become narrower.

Gonorrhoea

Signs and symptoms

It is possible to be infected with gonorrhoea and not have symptoms. Men are far more likely to notice symptoms than women. Gonorrhoea is a type of bacteria.

Women

Symptoms can include:
- a change in vaginal discharge. This may increase, change to a yellow or greenish colour and develop a strong smell
- a pain or burning sensation when passing urine
- irritation and/or discharge from the anus.

Men

Symptoms may include:
- a yellow or white discharge from the penis
- irritation and/or discharge from the anus
- inflammation of the testicles and prostate gland.

Transmission

Gonorrhoea is passed on through:
- penetrative sex.

And less often by:
- inserting your fingers into an infected vagina, anus or mouth and then putting them into your own without washing your hands in between
- sharing vibrators or other sex toys.

Diagnosis and treatment

Samples are taken, using a swab, from any area that may be infected—the cervix, urethra, anus or throat. A sample of urine may be taken. If the tests are positive, antibiotics can be given.

Long-term effects

If left untreated gonorrhoea can lead to pelvic inflammatory disease in women. This can cause fever, pain and can lead to infertility or ectopic pregnancy.

A woman can pass it on to her baby if she is infected when the baby is born.

In men, gonorrhoea can cause inflammation of the testicles and the prostate gland, which causes pain. Without treatment the urethra may become narrower.

Genital herpes

Signs and symptoms

Both men and women may have one or more symptoms, including:
- an itching or tingling sensation in the genital or anal area
- small fluid-filled blisters. These burst and leave small sores that can be painful. In time they dry out, scab over and heal. The first infection can take between two and four weeks to heal
- pain when passing urine, if it passes over any of the open sores
- a flu-like illness, backache, headache, swollen glands or fever (at this time, the virus is highly infectious)
- recurrent infections are usually milder. The sores are fewer, smaller, less painful and heal more quickly.

Genital herpes affects both men and women and is caused by a virus.

Transmission

Herpes is passed on through direct contact with an infected person. The virus affects the areas where it enters the body. This can be by:
- penetrative sex (when the penis enters the vagina, mouth or anus)
- oral sex (from mouth to the genitals).

Diagnosis and treatment
- A clinical examination of the genital area is carried out by a doctor or a nurse.
- A sample is taken, using a cotton-wool swab, from any visible sores.

Tablets can reduce the severity of the infection; these are only effective when taken within 72 hours of the start of the symptoms. A cream is available to control the symptoms. Recurrent infections may not need treatment.

During an episode of herpes, the blisters and sores are highly infectious and the virus can be passed on to others by direct contact. To prevent this from happening, the following should be avoided:
- oral sex when there are mouth or genital sores
- any genital or anal contact, even with a condom or dental dam, when there are genital sores
- sharing of towels and face flannels.

Long-term effects

Having herpes does not affect a woman's ability to become pregnant, but if herpes occurs in the first three months of pregnancy there is a small risk of miscarriage.

If an individual has an episode of herpes when the baby is due, they may be advised to have a caesarean delivery to reduce the risk of infecting the baby.

Genital warts

(Human papillomavirus)
Signs and symptoms

- Pinkish/white small lumps or larger cauliflower-shaped lumps on the genital area.
- Warts on the vulva, penis, scrotum or anus, in the vagina and on the cervix.
- It usually takes one to three months from infection for warts to appear.
- Warts may itch but are usually painless.
- Not everyone who comes into contact with the virus will develop warts.

Transmission

Warts are spread through skin-to-skin contact therefore can be caught through genital contact as well as sexual intercourse.

Diagnosis and treatment

A doctor or nurse can usually diagnose genital warts by looking. An internal examination may be carried out to check for warts in the vagina or anus. A common treatment for genital warts is to paint on a liquid called podophyllin. They can also be treated by freezing or laser treatment.

   If you have genital warts you should also:

- keep the genital area clean and dry
- not use scented soaps, bath oils or vaginal deodorants
- use condoms when having sex—these will protect against warts only if they cover the affected area
- make sure your partner has a check-up too.

Long-term effects

Most people will have recurrence of warts that will need further treatment. Some types of the wart virus may be linked to changes in cervical cells that can lead to cervical cancer. It is important that all women over 25 years of age have a regular cervical smear test.

Additional resources

NHS Cervical Screening Programme

To find out more, go to the following website:

www.cancerscreening.nhs.uk/cervical/index.html

THE HUMAN PAPILLOMA VIRUS (HPV) OR 'WART VIRUS' VACCINE

The wart virus has been in the news a lot recently. About a year ago a national immunisation programme was introduced to vaccinate year eight girls against some forms of HPV virus as it can reduce the occurrence of cervical cancer in future years. This caused much debate. As it was to be done before young people were sexually active some felt that it might encourage them to have sexual intercourse earlier or without protection as they may feel that they have been protected against STIs generally by the vaccine. Neither of these need be true. It has been proven that general sexual health promotion and sex and relationship education do not lead to young people having sex earlier, it simply means they are better informed if and when they do. Also, with the correct information given alongside the HPV vaccine young women should be aware that the vaccine protects against one STI only.

In addition, Jade Goody's death from cervical cancer has led a national debate on whether the age of the first cervical screening should be brought back to 20 rather than 25, where it currently stands. It was moved because a woman's cervix at age 20 is still growing and changing; the tests were also looking for cells that were changing and might lead to precancerous cells. The outcome was that many women had a lot of unnecessary investigations, with the related stress and anxiety. However, since then the method of screening has changed, becoming more accurate in sampling and reading.

Certainly the media coverage of Jade Goody has led to an increased demand for cervical screening from those under the age of 25. Should these women have to wait until they are 25, or with the right counselling, should they be able to access cervical screening from the age of 20?

Print out the following information about the vaccine; this can be used to instigate debate with your group.

How do they feel about it?

Should boys be having it too?

Do they think it will make young people more likely to start having sex earlier, or without using a condom?

Do they have any concerns?

Schoolgirls to get 'cancer jab'

From September 2008 schoolgirls in Britain have been vaccinated against the virus that causes cervical cancer.

It is thought that vaccinating against human papilloma virus (HPV) could save hundreds of lives in the UK each year. It will prevent up to 85% of cervical cancers.

The vaccine is given in three injections over six months at a cost of around £300 a course.

The programme will be offered to girls aged 12 to 13.

Some have expressed concerns that providing a jab to protect against a sexually transmitted infection to children at a young age might encourage promiscuity. The aim is to provide immunity before sexual activity commences.

About 80% of sexually active women can expect to have an HPV infection at some point in their lives. It is held responsible for some 70% of cervical cancer cases, a disease which kills 274 000 women worldwide every year, including 1 120 in the UK.

Invite a school health nurse to speak to your group about cervical cancer, the screening programme and the HPV vaccine.

Use the following handout to stimulate debate about cervical screening and at what age the screening programme should start.

Should the age of first cervical screening be lowered?

Cervical cancer is extremely rare in women younger than 25. Cases of cervical cancer in women under 25 make up just 1.7% of all cases in women under the age of 70 in the UK.

Women in Scotland, Wales and Northern Ireland are offered smear tests from the age of 20. Yet many European countries start at the same age as us or later, including Belgium, France, Ireland and Italy. The Netherlands and Finland don't begin screening until the age of 30.

Evidence has shown that smoking and having unprotected sex at an earlier age can increase the risk of developing cervical abnormalities. These lifestyle choices are becoming increasingly common among younger women, and teenage girls' screening should begin at a younger age.

Women in England used to be invited for cervical screening at age 20 but in 2003 the threshold was raised to 25. The reasoning behind the decision was based on research on the negative effects of testing young women.

Natural changes to the cervix are common in women under 25: this is because at this age, young women's bodies are still developing. If under 25s are screened, many of these harmless changes will be detected and give a false-positive result, causing unnecessary concern for many young women. Further investigation into these cases could cause more harm than good, with testing procedures causing discomfort and the removal of cervical tissue, increasing the risk of premature birth in the future.

It can be argued that the NHS has set this threshold for economic reasons. There is no doubt it is a more cost-effective strategy than investigating thousands of false-positive cases.

How is HPV related to cervical cancer?

- Some types of HPV can infect a woman's cervix and cause the cells to change.
- Most of the time, HPV goes away.
- Sometimes it persists and continues to change the cells.
- These cell changes can lead to cancer over time if they are not treated.
- About 3 000 women are diagnosed with this type of cancer every year in the UK.

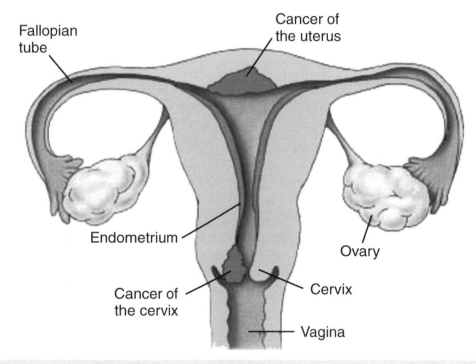

Figure 10.1 Cervical cancer

How common is HPV?

- At least 50% of sexually active people will get HPV at some time in their lives.

How will a vaccine help?

- It protects against four HPV types.
- These types cause 70% of cervical cancers and 90% of genital warts.

What does the vaccine *not* protect against?

- As the vaccine does not protect against *all* types of HPV, it will not prevent all cases of cervical cancer or genital warts.
- About 30% of cervical cancers will *not* be prevented by the vaccine, so it will be important for women to continue getting screened for cervical cancer (via regular smear tests).

- The vaccine does *not* prevent about 10% of genital warts.
- It will not prevent other sexually transmitted infections (STIs).

Who will be having it?

- The HPV vaccine is for 12 to 13 year old girls.
- It will also be offered to young women up to the age of 18 as a catch-up.

What about vaccinating boys?

- It is not yet known if the vaccine is effective in boys or men.
- It is possible that vaccinating males will have health benefits for them by preventing genital warts and cancers.
- Vaccinating boys/men may have indirect health benefits for girls/women
- Studies are now being done on males.
- When more information is available, this vaccine may be licensed and recommended for boys/men as well.

Why is the HPV vaccine recommended for such young girls?

- Ideally, females should get the vaccine before they are sexually active.
- The vaccine is most effective in girls/women who have not yet acquired any of the four HPV types covered by the vaccine.

How is the vaccine given?

- The HPV vaccine is given through a series of three injections over a six-month period.
- The second and third doses should be given two and six months after the first dose.

How long does vaccine protection last? Will a booster be needed?

- The length of vaccine protection is usually not known when a vaccine is first introduced.
- So far, studies have followed women for five years and found that women are still protected.
- More research is being done to find out how long protection will last, and whether a booster vaccine is needed years later.

Are there any side effects?

- This vaccine has been tested in over 11 000 females (ages 9 to 26 years) around the world. These studies have shown no serious side effects.

Additional resources

For more information on the HPV immunisation programme, see the following website:
www.nhs.uk/conditions/HPV-vaccination

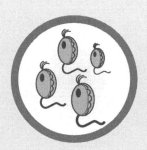

Trichomonas vaginalis (TV)

Signs and symptoms

Often trichomonas vaginalis has no symptoms, but in men and women discharge can occur along with genital soreness, pain when passing urine and pain during sex. Trichomonas vaginalis is a protozoan.

Diagnosis and treatment

Swabs from the vagina will be taken. Swabs are examined under the microscope and cultured. Women may be given an internal pelvic examination and men may have an external examination of their testicles and scrotum. Antibiotics easily treat TV.

Long-term effects

Complications associated with TV are rare.

Thrush, bacterial vaginosis and cystitis

Thrush, bacterial vaginosis and cystitis are not necessarily sexually transmitted. Whilst they can occur through other means independently of sexual intercourse, they are included here as sex can precipitate these conditions. Sexual intercourse can alter the pH of the vagina where thrush and bacterial vaginosis can colonise. Sex can also introduce bacteria to the urethra in men and women causing cystitis.

Thrush

Thrush is caused by a yeast that normally lives harmlessly on the skin, or in the mouth, gut and vagina without causing any problems. Usually it is kept in check by harmless bacteria. Occasionally conditions change and the yeast increases rapidly, causing symptoms.

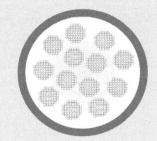

Sexual transmission is thought to play a limited part in the epidemiology of thrush. Antibiotics given for other conditions can cause thrush to develop.

Signs and symptoms
Women:
- itching, soreness and redness around the vagina, vulva or anus
- a thick, white discharge from the vagina that looks like cottage cheese and smells yeasty
- a swollen vulva
- pain when you have sex or pass urine.

Men:
- irritation, burning or itching under the foreskin or on the tip of the penis
- a redness, or red patches, under the foreskin or on the tip of the penis
- a thick, cheesy discharge under the foreskin
- difficulty in pulling back the foreskin
- a slight discharge from the urethra
- discomfort when passing urine.

There is an increased chance of developing thrush with the following:
- wearing lycra shorts or tight nylon clothes
- taking certain antibiotics
- using too much vaginal deodorant or perfumed bubble bath, causing irritation
- having sex with someone who has a thrush infection
- diabetes.

Diagnosis and treatment
Thrush can be diagnosed by:
- an examination of the genital area by a doctor or a nurse
- samples are taken using swabs for close examination under a microscope.

A cream is applied to the external genital area, and women may be given pessaries to insert into the vagina using a special applicator. Oral anti-thrush tablets are also available. These treatments are available from chemists.

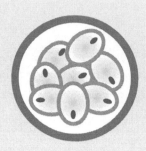

Bacterial vaginosis

Bacterial vaginosis (BV) is a common infection of the vagina. Bacterial vaginosis is the commonest cause of abnormal vaginal discharge in women of childbearing age. It is twice as common as vaginal thrush.

Signs and symptoms
These include vaginal discharge that is white-grey in colour and fishy smelling.

Diagnosis and treatment
BV is not caused by a single type of bacteria, it is an overgrowth of various bacteria in the vagina. BV is not caused by poor hygiene; in fact, excessive washing of the vagina may alter the normal balance of the bacteria in the vagina, which may make BV more likely to develop. A nurse or doctor may take a vaginal swab that can be looked at under the microscope and observe the vaginal area for discharge and characteristic fishy smell.

BV is self-limiting; however, it can also be easily treated with antibiotics. To prevent recurrences the following are also recommended:

- no vaginal douching
- no added bath oils, detergents or bubble bath to bath water
- not washing around the vaginal area too often.

Complications
BV during pregnancy is thought to cause some cases of early labour, miscarriage and uterine infection after childbirth. Antibiotic treatment is usually advised if BV occurs during pregnancy. If a client has BV the chances of developing a uterine infection following certain operations, e.g. termination of pregnancy, are higher. Therefore, antibiotics are given before various operations of the uterus if BV is diagnosed.

Cystitis (Urinary Tract Infection)

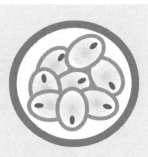

The commonest age to present with bacterial urinary tract infection (UTI) symptoms as an adult is around the mid-20s. Thirty-six per cent of women suffer a recurrence of symptoms within one year and 75% within 2 years. In 80% of cases the recurrence is due to a reinfection. A UTI is an extremely common reason for a visit to a general practitioner, accounting for between 1–6% of consultations.

Vaginal intercourse has an effect on susceptibility to UTIs, although the exact mechanism remains unknown. Episodes of cystitis are often associated with the onset of sexual intercourse, and women having regular intercourse have three to four times as many episodes of infection per year compared to women not having intercourse.

Signs and symptoms
Cystitis may cause one or more of the following symptoms:
- a burning feeling in the urethra on urination—sometimes there can be blood in the urine or it may be cloudy
- needing to pass water very frequently, even when little urine is present
- a dragging ache in the lower back or abdomen.

Cystitis can be caused by:
- bacteria—from the bowel
- friction—during sex
- 'irritable bladder'—a particularly sensitive bladder.

Diagnosis and treatment
There are over-the-counter treatments for cystitis from pharmacists. There are several 'home remedies' that can alleviate the symptoms:
- drinking lots of water (or any other bland liquid) to flush out bacteria and dilute the urine so that it does not sting as much when urinating
- taking a teaspoon of bicarbonate of soda mixed with half a pint of water, or other bland liquid, every hour. This makes the urine less acidic and stops bacteria multiplying. It also eases the stinging sensation when passing urine
- taking painkillers
- some women find that regular drinking of cranberry juice can help clear up an attack.

If symptoms persist the clinician will need a sample of urine to find out whether there is an infection and antibiotics are required.

How to avoid cystitis:
- always wipe your bottom from front to back
- drink plenty of bland fluids
- avoid perfumed products in the genital area
- wash and pass water before and after sex.

Infestations

Infestations occur where there is skin-to-skin contact, therefore they are associated with sexual intercourse.

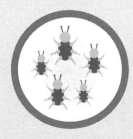

Pubic lice

The exact incidence of pubic lice is unknown, but it is thought to be quite common among young adults.

Signs and symptoms

The most common symptom is itching in the infected areas, and it may be possible to see droppings from the lice in underwear (black powder) as well as eggs on pubic or other hair. It is sometimes possible to see lice on the skin.

Transmission

Pubic lice are usually sexually transmitted but can occasionally be transferred by close physical contact or by sharing sheets or towels.

Diagnosis and treatment

The lice can be detected by physical examination and may be examined under a microscope. Special shampoo or lotion can easily treat the lice. Any partners of the infected person should be treated.

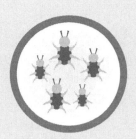

Scabies

Scabies has a cyclical rise in incidence roughly every 20 years in the UK. Reported cases have risen in the UK since 1991, often presenting as outbreaks in schools and residential or nursing homes. Scabies is more prevalent in urban than rural areas, and in winter than in summer. Scabies is more prevalent in children and young adults, but all ages can be affected.

Signs and symptoms

The main symptom of scabies is an itchy rash on hands, wrists, elbows, underneath the arms, and on the abdomen, breasts, genitals and buttocks.

Transmission

Scabies is not necessarily sexually transmitted as any close physical contact can spread the infection.

Diagnosis and treatment

The rash can be seen on physical examination and may be examined under a microscope. Scabies is easily treated by special shampoo or lotion.

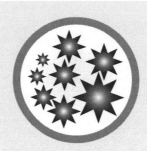

HIV and AIDS

Human immunodeficiency virus (HIV) is the virus that causes acquired immunodeficiency syndrome (AIDS). AIDS is a serious condition in which the body's defences against some illnesses are broken down. This means that people with AIDS are vulnerable to many different diseases which a healthy person's body would normally deal with quite easily.

There is still no cure for HIV; however, medication to offset the complications of the disease are increasingly available and in forms and regimes that are easier to take. Since treatment to offset the complications of the illness are readily available, young people are encouraged to take the test. If they are positive, they can have a nigh on normal life expectancy with less illness if the condition is diagnosed early on.

How long does it take for HIV to cause AIDS?
The length of time between being infected with HIV and being diagnosed with AIDS depends on many things. Currently there are drugs that can be used to offset the development of AIDS from HIV.

How do you get infected?
HIV is passed on via sexual fluids or the blood of an infected person. This usually happens through sexual intercourse with an infected person or by sharing needles with an infected person. Mothers may pass HIV to a child at childbirth (HIV can also be passed through breast milk), and a very small number of people become infected by having medical treatment using infected blood transfusions.

Oral sex carries some risk of infection. Infected fluid could get into the mouth, where the virus enters into the blood via bleeding gums or sores. Infection from oral sex alone is very rare.

How can I get tested?
HIV is detected via a blood test. It is advisable to wait three months after the last risky sexual contact before having the test. This is because the virus is not detectable before this 'window period'.

Brook Advisory Centre

Helpline: 0800 0185 023 (Monday to Thursdays 9 a.m.–5 p.m., Fridays 9 a.m.–4 p.m.)
Website: www.brook.org.uk

Provides free and confidential contraceptive advice for anyone under 25. Provides emergency contraception, pregnancy testing and counselling on any sex and relationship problem. Offers 24-hour recorded messages on pregnancy, contraception, abortion and sexually transmitted diseases: 0207 617 8000.

Additional resources

AVERT

Information for young people about HIV infection and AIDS, sex, puberty, sexuality, contraception and condoms. Includes personal stories, articles and resources such as quizzes, statistics, FAQs and printable booklets. www.avert.org

Family Planning Association (FPA)

Leaflets on STIs are available on their website at www.fpa.org.uk

Virtual tour of a sexual health clinic

www.thesite.org/audioandvideo/video/sexandrelationships/gumclinicvirtualtour

NHS Choices videos

'The Chlamydia Test'

A dramatisation of a teenage couple, Ben and Rosie, going for tests for STIs including chlamydia is available at:
http://tinyurl.com/yf7j6mm

'Teens and STIs'

How to find out if you have an STI, how it can be treated, and how it can affect young people's health:
http://tinyurl.com/ydyq9td

CHAPTER 11

L8r baby!
Teenage pregnancy

Teenage pregnancy is a hot issue. It has been identified by the government as an area that needs particular attention. The government has actually set up a specific department, the Teenage Pregnancy Unit, to identify and deal with issues pertaining to teen pregnancy.

It is commonly thought with the coverage and publicity that teenage pregnancy receives that it is statistically the worst it has ever been in England and Wales. It is true we do not compare favourably with neighbouring European countries, yet in fact the statistics have been steadily improving since the 1970s. This has been put down to the increased availability of contraception, the introduction of the abortion act in 1967 which increased the availability of legal abortion, and a heightened awareness of sexual health and contraceptive issues amongst the population as a whole.

Despite the statistics, teenagers are in fact far less likely to get pregnant today than they were in the early 1970s. The decline in teenage motherhood is even more striking. The proportion of pregnant teenagers choosing motherhood declined sharply after the 1967 Abortion Act offered young people the choice of terminating an unwanted pregnancy.

In previous centuries people generally married younger and child bearing was traditionally reserved for marriage. As times have changed adolescence is associated with being a time for education, and achieving financial and social independence prior to forming relationships. Having children during this time could be seen as interrupting and hindering achievement in these areas, and making it difficult to achieve in the future.

In addition, young parents can find it difficult to finish their education and/ or find and hold down a job. This leaves them socially isolated and at a financial disadvantage. The government has labelled this 'social exclusion' and it is this, rather than teenage pregnancy per se, that they want to avoid.

Other factors

In addition there are health consequences for young parents and their children. Pregnant teens often do not seek and/or get adequate prenatal care, missing out on important scans and blood tests as well as possible support networks. Children of teens are at increased risk of low birth-weight babies, infant mortality, sudden infant death syndrome, and increased rates of illness and injury.

WHAT IS KNOWN TO INFLUENCE TEENAGE PREGNANCY?

Education

There is a clear link between education and teen pregnancy rates. The level of education is inversely proportional to numbers of teen pregnancies; the higher the level of education, the less teen pregnancy. This appears to be for two reasons: young people who don't see themselves going on in education will not feel they have lost any opportunities by becoming young parents, and once a young person becomes pregnant the chances of her completing her education are greatly reduced. Despite good intentions it can be difficult to combine a highly timetabled school life with a not-so-timetabled child. It is difficult for schools to be flexible, and the struggle to combine motherhood and education can deter young people from continuing their schooling. Moreover, if teen mothers fail to stay in school there is a greater chance for a closer-spaced subsequent birth. Therefore poor academic performance is considered a determinant and consequence of childbearing too early.

Poverty

Nationally, the risk of becoming a teenage mother is almost 10 times higher for a girl whose family is in social class V (unskilled manual), than those in social class I (professional). Once a young woman has become a teenage parent it is difficult to finish education and/or find and hold down a job and establish independence from family and state. This perpetuates the poverty cycle. There is an increased chance of becoming a teenage mother if a young woman's own mother had a teen pregnancy.

Many teenage mothers have family support. Seven out of ten 15 and 16 year olds and half 17 and 18 year olds stay in their parental home with their child. This has psychological as well as monetary benefits for the young person, as she is likely to have help with childcare and be more able to return to school or work. It does, however, put financial pressure on the extended family.

Motivation

There is a general assumption that teen pregnancy is accidental. It appears to be a teenager's failure to understand her risk, inability to obtain contraception, or inability to negotiate contraceptive use with her partner that have led to her becoming pregnant. Yet this makes the assumption that all teenage girls are motivated to prevent pregnancy. In fact some teens may consciously want to become pregnant or simply may not mind being pregnant. They may see pregnancy as a means of achieving adulthood, finding a purpose in life, having someone to love and strengthening their relationship with their sexual partner.

When young people do not have academic nor employment aspirations, lost opportunities through having a child will not be a consideration. Consequently they are more likely to engage in unprotected sex, or be less committed to avoiding pregnancy, or actively seek parenthood.

Family and friends

Friends are more likely to be consulted by pregnant teens at the beginning of a pregnancy, yet family members are more important in finalising the teens' decision. Family members and friends can directly influence a young person's choices regarding childbearing. They may actively encourage childbearing or abortion if a young person is faced with the choice of whether to keep a pregnancy. Young people will have also observed the choices people have made around them regarding childbearing, which will in turn influence their own choices. A young woman may be influenced for or against having a baby by whether or not her friends have babies and whether she has seen these friends have positive or negative experiences.

Partner

A young woman's partner can influence her decision to become pregnant or not and her decision once pregnant. He can encourage her to keep the baby as an expression of their love, or put pressure on to have an abortion. It is important to recognise that he is often directly involved in the decision and his influence should be considered when the young women's decisions are being discussed. The couple may not necessarily be in a long-term, committed relationship. One study has shown that only half of teen mothers are still in a relationship with the father a year after the baby's birth; the other half have no steady partner. Hence the father is often distanced from the consequences of teen pregnancy and is less likely to feel responsible for preventing pregnancy in the future.

SO WHAT CAN WE DO?

What is different about countries that have low teen pregnancy rates? They have similar social class variations, education levels and areas of poverty, however the differences appear to lie in the following areas:
- they have an open and accepting attitude to teenage sexuality
- they offer widely available information and sex education
- there is easy access to confidential contraceptive services.

For the professional working with young people, a holistic approach to the sexual health of young people is required. This would include access to accurate and up-to-date information on contraception, abortion and pregnancy, and knowledge of local services providing for young people's sexual health and contraception, pregnancy and counselling. Equally vital is having an accepting attitude to young people's sexuality, being willing to talk about sex, raising a young person's self-esteem, and encouraging her ambition and life goals when teen pregnancy would be an obstacle.

Prevention work

Prevention work is essential; the ideal would be that all young people delay sexual activity. This would reduce teenage pregnancy and the prevalence of STIs as well as the psychological impact of early sexual relationships. However, it is not enough to simply tell young people not to have sex. In a society where they are constantly surrounded by sexual images, an abstinence message can be confusing and counterproductive. It can result in the perpetuation of myths and misinformation about sex and contraception amongst young people, leading to an increase in unintentional risk-taking behaviour; young people find themselves in a relationship and do not have the knowledge or skills to negotiate boundaries and prevent STIs and pregnancy. In fact, it has been found that if young people have clear and accurate information regarding sex and contraception before they begin to explore their sexuality, they delay sexual activity. In addition, young people are more likely to practice safe sex when they do become sexually active.

Sex education that includes discussion of the emotional aspects of relationships with role-playing is helpful in strengthening young people's assertiveness over relationship issues and contraception use. Negotiation skills in relationships should be incorporated into any work on sexual health with young people. Negotiation skills are an important part of the SRE curriculum, but are useful skills in all areas of life; also important are a raised awareness of how sex and sexuality are used in the media and the encouragement of critical awareness regarding such tactics.

PREGNANCY

The main aims within this subject are to give young people the knowledge of how pregnancy happens, how they can avoid becoming pregnant, the impact of having children, and the choices available to them if they do become pregnant.

Pregnancy and parenting

How does pregnancy happen?

- Pregnancy occurs when a sperm reaches the egg and joins on to it; this is called fertilisation. This can happen when two people have sex and do not use contraception or, in rare cases, when the chosen method of contraception fails.

How do I reduce my risk of pregnancy?

Although contraceptives offer excellent protection against pregnancy when used properly, no method is 100% effective.

- Always practice safer sex by using a condom.
- Always read the instructions carefully for the method of contraception you have chosen to use.
- Never presume you are not at risk from becoming pregnant, regardless of the stage of your menstrual cycle.
- Abstinence is the only way you can be sure you won't get pregnant.

How do I know if I'm pregnant?

- Your period may be late and you may suffer any of the following: nausea and vomiting, fatigue, headaches, increased urine production, discomfort passing water, enlarged and painful breasts and nipples, and your temperature may rise a little.

How can I find out if I'm pregnant?

- If you suspect that you are pregnant, your first step is to take a pregnancy test and seek medical advice.

How will I be tested?

- A urine or blood sample may be taken by a medical professional, along with an examination to confirm whether you are pregnant. Some pharmacies offer home pregnancy testing kits you can use yourself. A negative result means you are not pregnant and a positive result means that you are pregnant.

Who can I talk to?
- You can talk it over with your partner or your parents. If you don't feel you can talk to them you could speak to an older brother or sister, friends, a teacher, a doctor or nurse. Remember to seek information from an impartial source. It is also important to make the right decision for you.

What are my choices?
- Continue the pregnancy and keep the baby.
- Continue the pregnancy and place the baby for adoption.
- End the pregnancy by having an abortion.

How will having a baby affect my life?
- Having a baby will affect you physically, emotionally, socially and financially, and you will have responsibility for the child for the rest of your life.

A young woman may come to you, a trusted adult, for advice; the following information could be given to the young person to think through on her own, or it could be used as a prompt in your discussion with her.

Unplanned pregnancy choices

What are my choices?
- Continue the pregnancy and keep the baby.
- Continue the pregnancy and place the baby for adoption.
- End the pregnancy by having an abortion.

How can I decide which choice is best for me?
Consider each of your choices carefully. Ask yourself:
- which choice(s) could I live with?
- which choice(s) would be impossible for me?
- how would each choice affect my everyday life?
- what would each choice mean to the people closest to me?

It may also help to ask yourself:
- what is going on in my life?
- how does my current boyfriend feel about this?
- what are my plans for the future?
- what are my spiritual and moral beliefs?
- what do I believe is best for me in the long run?
- what can I afford?

What should I do while I decide?

While you are deciding what to do, take good care of yourself. If you decide to have a child, it's important to be healthy. You should:

- eat enough good food—fruits, vegetables, cereals, breads, beans, rice, and dairy products, as well as fish, meat and poultry
- keep your body in good shape. Stay active and get regular exercise such as walking and swimming
- get plenty of sleep
- do not smoke
- do not drink alcohol and reduce drinks with caffeine
- do not eat junk food
- do not take any drugs or medications without checking with your clinician or doctor.

You can get complete information about antenatal care from your family doctor or contraception clinics. Good antenatal care is very important for a baby's health.

 Use the following role plays to explore scenarios around pregnancy. These could be done in pairs simultaneously, with each pair feeding back the issues that come out of the activity to the wider group. Alternatively they could be done in front of the group, with comments and discussion from the group after the role play.

A girl finds out that she is pregnant and decides to tell her parents

A girl finds out that she is pregnant and decides to tell her boyfriend

A girl thinks she may be pregnant and asks her best friend for advice

A boy finds out that his girlfriend is pregnant and asks his best friend for advice

A mother/father discovers a home pregnancy test in their daughter's bedroom

A pregnant girl and her boyfriend discuss the options available to them

Your boyfriend says the baby is not his

ADOPTION

There have been far fewer children placed for adoption in recent years. The rapid decline in the number of children available for adoption followed the introduction of legal abortion in the Abortion Act 1967 and the implementation of the Children Act 1975. The latter Act gave the court power to treat an adoption application as an application for a custodianship order if the court considered this to be in the child's best interests.

In December 2005, the Adoption and Children Act 2002 was fully implemented. It replaced the Adoption Act 1976 and modernised the legal framework for adoption in England and Wales. The Act provides for an adoption order to be made in favour of single people, married couples and, for the first time, civil partners, same-sex couples and unmarried couples. The Act also introduced Special Guardianship to provide permanence for children who cannot return to their birth families, but for whom adoption is not the most suitable option.

Adoption

Some people may decide that they could continue the pregnancy without bringing up the child.

What is adoption?
- Adoption is the legal process of giving up responsibility for your child.

How does the adoption process work?
- The courts will ensure that you are definite about your decision to place the baby up for adoption (unless the baby is going to a family member) and that the baby's new home is the right environment for him/her to grow up in.

Are there different kinds of adoption?
- *Closed adoption*—the names of the birth mother and the adoptive parents are kept secret from each other.
- *Open adoption*—the birth mother may select the adoptive parents for her child. She and the adoptive parents may choose to get to know each other. They may also choose to have an ongoing relationship.

How is adoption arranged?
Adoption is arranged in three ways:
- *agency (licensed) adoption*—the birth parents 'relinquish' their child to the agency. The agency places the child into the adoptive home
- *independent (unlicensed) adoption*—the birth parents relinquish their child directly into the adoptive home
- *adoption by relatives*—the court grants legal adoption to relatives.

What if I change my mind?
- The adoption process is usually made legal three months after the birth, up to this point you are free to change your mind.
- Many women who make this choice are happy knowing their children are loved and living in good homes. But some women find that the pain of being separated from their child is deeper and longer lasting than they expected.

What's the difference between adoption and fostering?
- Fostering means that another set of parents will temporarily look after your child but you remain the legal guardian and will hopefully be in a position to care for your child in the future.

ABORTION

Abortion is a subject from which professionals seem to shy away. It is a subject that can invoke strong feelings and beliefs both from the person facilitating a session and those participating in it. It is often seen as a sensitive topic and one that may offend people of certain beliefs or culture.

However, young people are entitled to have unbiased, accurate information about their health so they can make informed decisions. Research shows that the majority of young women experiencing unintended pregnancy have not considered their pregnancy options in advance of their pregnancy. As a result they are most likely to be guided in their choices by socio-economic factors or family and cultural expectations, rather than consideration of how having a child or another child fits into their lives. For a young man who experiences an unplanned pregnancy with a partner, it is important that he knows who he can talk to and where he can go for help and support, as well as being able to signpost his partner to appropriate agencies.

Exploring the subject of abortion with your group/young person can be an opportunity to reinforce the importance of consensual, mutual and safe relationships, within which safer sex practices can be negotiated and agreed. Covering the efficacy and availability of contraception and signposting to sources of confidential contraceptive advice and treatment are cornerstones of effective abortion education.

Abortion education helps young people to develop the vocabulary, confidence and skills they need to be able to talk to parents, carers, and health professionals about sex relationships, contraception, pregnancy and abortion.

THE LAW

Two doctors must sign a certificate stating that the woman satisfies the legal criteria for abortion.

It is notable that approximately 10% of GPs will not refer women for abortion because they oppose abortion in principle. The law allows doctors to opt out of providing or participating in abortions if their conscience prevents them from doing so. However, most medical bodies advise that a doctor should help a woman by telling her where to go in order to get a referral, even if he will not refer her himself.

Grounds for abortion

Grounds for an abortion under the (United Kingdom) 1967 Abortion Act as amended under section 37 of the Human and Embryology Act 1990.

Please note: Although there was an upper time limit of 24 weeks brought in by the 1990 amendment, this only applies to Grounds C and D. All other Grounds are without time limit, which means that these abortions can be carried out up to birth.

A	The continuance of the pregnancy would involve risk to the life of the pregnant woman greater than if the pregnancy were terminated;
B	The termination is necessary to prevent grave permanent injury to the physical or mental health of the pregnant woman;
C	The continuance of the pregnancy would involve risk, greater than if the pregnancy were terminated, of injury to the physical or mental health of the pregnant woman;
D	The continuance of the pregnancy would involve risk, greater than if the pregnancy were terminated, of injury to the physical or mental health of any existing child(ren) of the family of the pregnant woman;
E	There is a substantial risk that if the child were born it would suffer from such physical or mental abnormalities as to be seriously handicapped
F	To save the life of the pregnant woman; or
G	To prevent grave permanent injury to the physical or mental health of the pregnant woman.

Abortion methods

Consultant gynaecologists who oversee abortion can decide which methods of abortion they prefer to be used at different stages of pregnancy. Depending on the gestation of the pregnancy (which is calculated by counting from the first day of the woman's last menstrual period) and the preference of the doctor, women are sometimes given a choice about the abortion method and the form of anaesthetic used. Most abortions take place within the first 12 weeks of pregnancy, when one of two methods will be used:

Early medical abortion
- Typically used up to nine weeks gestation.
- Two appointments: one where tablets are given, and one two days later where the products of conception are passed through the cervix. Drugs are used to cause an early miscarriage. One works by blocking the action of the hormone that makes the lining of the uterus hold onto the fertilised egg. The other, given 48 hours later, causes the uterus to cramp. The lining of the uterus breaks down and the embryo is lost in the bleeding that follows. There will be some pain, like period pain. There will be some bleeding, which can be irregular and last a while.

Vacuum aspiration abortion

- Typically used between five and 15 weeks gestation.
- Requires attendance at a hospital or licenced premises for half a day.
- Vacuum aspiration is another term for suction. During vacuum aspiration abortion a thin, round-ended plastic tube is eased into the uterus through the cervix and attached to a pump. The contents of the uterus are then suctioned away through the tube. It is possible to have a vacuum aspiration abortion under a local or a general anaesthetic and the procedure takes about 10 minutes to perform.
- With a local anaesthetic, which numbs the cervix, there will be some cramps, like period pain. If the woman has a general anaesthetic (i.e. she goes to sleep) she won't feel anything. After the abortion there may be some pain, like period pain, and bleeding, like a period. This can last up to 14 days.

Dilatation and evacuation

- Usually used between 14-19 weeks gestation.
- Usually requires one day at a clinic or hospital, and possibly an overnight stay.
- Narrow forceps remove the contents of the womb. Suction might also be used.
- This is carried out under general anaesthetic. There may be some pain afterwards and bleeding for up to 14 days.

Medical induction

- Usually used for gestation over 13 weeks.
- Usually requires one night in a clinic or hospital, though sometimes it can be done in a day.
- There are two methods. Most women are given pessaries to induce a miscarriage and may be given the abortion pill two days before they come into hospital. Some women have an injection into the womb instead of the pessaries.
- There may be some strong cramping pains. Afterwards there may be some pain, like period pain, and bleeding for about a week, though possibly longer.
- In later pregnancy, other abortion methods are available.

Frequently asked questions

Are there risks at the time of abortion or afterwards?

Problems at the time of abortion are not very common. As with any operation, the commonest risk is from infection. In many cases the infection is a flare-up of a pre-existing sexually transmitted infection such as chlamydia. Women will usually be checked for this before their abortion. There is an extremely small risk of damage to the womb. Repeated abortions, and abortions in later pregnancy, increase the risk, but all legal abortion methods are still very safe.

Will abortion affect a woman's chances of having a baby in the future?

There are no proven associations between induced abortion and subsequent ectopic pregnancy (where the pregnancy develops outside the womb) or infertility.

Does abortion cause breast cancer?

Having an abortion does not increase a woman's lifetime risk of developing breast cancer.

What will happen when you are referred to a termination of pregnancy (TOP) clinic?

There are usually two appointments.

The first appointment is where all the assessments take place. You will be asked general questions about your health, you will have blood tests for your blood type (a normal procedure for any operation in the rare case you need to be given blood), then you will be given a pelvic ultrasound scan to double check how pregnant you are and an explanation of the procedure and your consent is obtained.

For a surgical termination the second appointment will be when the actual procedure takes place. This will either be in morning or afternoon surgery. You will be able to go home once you feel OK after the anaesthetic has worn off. It is a good idea to have someone pick you up.

For a medical termination, taking the initial tablets to stop the pregnancy may happen at the assessment stage or at a different appointment. Two days later at a morning attendance at hospital or another licensed premises you will be given a vaginal tablet. This opens the cervix and allows the 'products of conception' to come out.

In both types, on very rare occasions, you may need to stay on in hospital.

This activity helps the group understand that before planning to have children, parents should have stability and prepare themselves physically, emotionally and financially.

Prepare lots of paper bricks and ask the young people to list the factors that can build a solid foundation to a relationship, and write these in the bricks.

Stick these up to form a wall, discussing as you go along.

Make a large 'wrecking ball'.

Get the young people to think of the things that can knock down that foundation and fill these issues into the wrecking ball.

The following true or false quiz could be handed out as a paper exercise or used as a prompt for group discussion.

Abortion

1 Most abortions in Britain are carried out early—in the first 12 weeks of pregnancy.
2 The law says that a doctor can provide advice and treatment (including abortion) to young people under the age of 16.
3 If you request an abortion, your GP is legally obliged to help you.
4 Giving birth is safer than having a legal abortion.
5 Women who choose to have an abortion can change their mind at any time.
6 Abortion is bad for your health.
7 Abortion is bad for your mental health.
8 The legal limit for abortion is 20 weeks in the UK.

The following scenario could be used as a prompt for group discussion. The group could be split into two, one taking the standpoint of the mother, and the other as the young woman; or even three to include the health professional. (This is a real life scenario.)

A 14-year-old girl had an abortion without her mother knowing. She accessed the abortion via a health worker at school. Her mum eventually found out, the young girl changed her mind, but it was too late by then as she had already taken the tablets for a medical termination. The young woman said she had the termination because she felt she had let her mum and dad down. Health workers are not legally bound to tell parents when a young woman is pregnant.

Directory of local contraception clinics

A leaflet called 'Abortion; just so you know' is available at: www.fpa.org.uk

Additional information
Evidence-based and patient information on abortion can be found at: www.rcog.org.uk

Additional resources

Confidential young people's sexual health clinics providing pregnancy decision-making support and referral for antenatal and abortion services can be found at: www.brook.org.uk

Information on benefits and support for young parents is listed at: www.oneparentfamilies.org

www.surestart.gov.uk

To access private abortion, call Actionline for advice: 08457 30 40 30

www.bpas.org.uk

www.mariestopes.org.uk

Helpline: 0845 300 8090

CHAPTER 12

Gangs

For the purpose of this chapter we will be focusing on the more antisocial and even criminal aspect of gangs. Our main aim is to understand the origin and nature of gang culture, to identify young people who may be at risk of becoming involved in gangs or are already involved, and to employ strategies to help young people avoid becoming involved or more deeply involved in gangs.

Gang culture appears to be growing in the UK. Within gangs young people are often carrying imitation or real firearms and knives, both for protection and as part of their image. When violence erupts, it gains a high profile in the press. For example the shooting of Charlene Ellis and Letisha Shakespeare in Aston in 2003 received a huge amount of media attention. These incidents and others have increased public concern about the escalating problems relating to gangs, violence and drugs that are prevalent across some of the most deprived inner-city neighbourhoods.

The main question is: are these isolated incidents or is there an increasing problem with gang-related violence? Statistics from the Centre for Social Justice give an idea of the issues related to youth crime and gangs.

Statistics

Muggings

- Four in every 10 muggings in Britain are committed by children under 16 years old.

Knives

- The most likely person to be carrying a knife is a boy aged between 14 and 19.

Guns

- In 2002 nearly half of all gang murders committed with firearms involved victims under the age of 18.

Punishment

- Every year an estimated 70 000 school-aged offenders enter the youth justice system.
- The total number of young offenders in custody has been above 2 500 every month since April 2000. Latest figures show that 1 504 of the young people held in custody are 16 years old or younger.
- An estimated 11% of all prisoners involved in serious assaults are children; this is despite accounting for just 3% of the general prison population.

Source: www.centreforsocialjustice.org.uk/default.asp?pageRef=214

WHAT IS A GANG?

Despite all the media attention to gangs we must be careful not to vilify all young people who are part of a group. Forming groups is a natural way for young people to identify with others away from the family unit, a way to learn to form relationships and participate in various interests. Not all groups of young people are antisocial and prone to committing crime!

Gangs often share an identity based either on age, location, ethnicity, peer networks or blood relationships and tend to be hierarchical communities with common interests and shared purposes.

Groups of young people have been categorised by the Jill Dando Institute (JDI). It is a useful tool for discriminating between the types of groups. The Institute identifies three groups:

Peer groups—Small, unorganized groups who share the same space and a common history. There will not be any criminal activity, or involvement in crime will mostly be at a low level and will not be important to the identity of the group.

Gangs—Mostly comprised of street-based groups of young people for whom crime and violence is an essential part of the group's identity. Groups tend to have a name.

Organised criminal groups—Groups of individuals for whom involvement in crime is for personal gain and is probably the individuals' main occupation. These groups operate in the illegal marketplace.

Have a discussion with the young people you work with about their perceptions of gangs. Do they feel under threat? Are they part of a gang? Do they think it is a problem or not?

Be very clear about confidentiality in this session, as revelation of involvement in crime will necessitate a breach of confidentiality.

HOW DO ORGANISED GANGS OPERATE?

Opinions vary as to levels of organisation within a gang. Research carried out in Manchester and Birmingham suggests that gangs consist of key individuals surrounded by ordinary members—the gang being more organised at the centre and less so on the edges, as follows:

Gang leaders—The leaders determine strategies and plan activities but do not get involved in committing offences.

Gang workers—These are established gang members caught up in the running of the business.

Foot soldiers—These are the youngest and most visible layer of a gang, and they are the most at risk of becoming victims of violent crime.

HOW VIOLENT ARE GANGS?

Once someone is a member of an organised gang it can be extremely difficult for him or her to leave, particularly when the gang feels that ex-members may divulge gang secrets or provide evidence against them to the police. Loyalty within a gang is so strong that members thought to have been disloyal are at risk of violence—even being killed.

There are links between gangs, guns and drugs, however this relationship is complicated. For instance, gang members are more likely than non-gang members to be drug dealers. Consequently, drug dealers may use firearms to protect themselves or enforce debts—yet it is important to highlight that not all gun crime is drug-related.

In addition, arrestee data shows that gang members are five times more likely than non-gang members to report owning a gun. One theory claims that a relationship may exist between the use of a weapon and the level of gang involvement—organised crime groups use guns whilst street gangs prefer knives. Being armed is partly protective, partly instrumental for engaging in violent crimes and partly symbolic.

WHO JOINS GANGS?

Despite wide variations in types of gangs and their activities, there are some common trends in gang structure and involvement. Gang members are predominately male, whilst females tend to follow gangs without becoming as heavily engaged in activity as their male counterparts—although there is anecdotal evidence that females may be starting to form their own gangs rather than seeking this approval through a member of a male gang. Females tend to be more involved in peer groups than street gangs.

Gangs may form due to social exclusion and discrimination—people come together for a sense of safety and belonging. Immigrant populations, those excluded from education or people who have engaged in criminal activities from an early age are particularly at risk of gang involvement. Others may join a gang simply for something to do, seeking protection in numbers, or for reasons of status and peer pressure.

Risk factors have been identified for young people joining a gang as the following.

- **Poverty**—A sense of hopelessness can result from being unable to purchase wanted goods and services. Young people living in poverty may find it difficult to meet basic physical and psychological needs, which can lead to a lack of self-worth and pride. One way to earn cash is to join a gang involved in the drug trade.
- **Lack of a support network**—Gang members often come from homes where they feel alienated or neglected. They may turn to gangs when their needs for love are not being met at home. Risks increase when the community fails to provide sufficient youth programmes or alternatives to violence.
- **Media influences**—Television, movies, radio and music all have profound effects on youth development. Before young people have established their own value systems and are able to make moral judgments, the media can promote drugs, sex and violence as an acceptable lifestyle.

- **Prejudice**—When young people encounter both personal and institutional prejudice (i.e. the systematic denial of privileges), the risks are increased. When groups of people are denied access to power, privileges, and resources, they will often form their own anti-establishment group.

'Youth Gangs: What's the attraction?'

Watch a video made by young people in west London looking at the issue of gangs. Discuss the issues raised.
www.headliners.org/storylibrary/stories/2008/youthgangs whatstheattraction.htm

The consequences of gang membership are never good—as the following video shows, the chances are higher that young people who get involved in gangs will be harmed or will harm someone and either end up dead or with a long prison sentence without much hope for the future.

Watch and discuss the issues raised in the excellent short film on YouTube called 'Killing don't get you nowhere', made by young people for young people with the support of The Fishing Rod Experience, the London Development Agency and the European Social Fund:
www.youtube.com/watch?v=GJUwO9zmaDc

Invite a case worker from the local youth offending team in to speak with the group about situations young people find themselves in, the consequences, and how to avoid these situations, and to answer the groups' questions on crime.

Print the following sheet and discuss the quotes with the young people in your group.
Put the quotes onto a notice board so discussion and awareness are maintained informally.

'I think what gangs offer you in comparison to a family are security and protection. Being in a gang means you always have someone watching your back, and people that feel they don't have that protection and support at home will look elsewhere for it.'

'There are many reasons why young people get into gangs. The main reason is just to have friends. Peer pressure can lead people into a situation where there is a need to feel like you belong to something. It can seem like a family, not all families are good though, but some are. It depends on what your gang does. You could be in a gang that helps old people across the road. A youth club is a gang, but not a negative one.'

'A friend of mine is in prison. He's older than me but he's in a gang and he's still got that gang mentality. I managed to get out, but he stayed in, and now he's in prison for stabbing someone and really truly it was over nothing, it was over a status. The guy said 'oh I'm badder than you, he's badder than you', so he stabbed him. Now that's it. His life is screwed up, if he comes out now he can't get a job, he can't have a proper life; he's going to be trapped for the rest of his life.'

'Gangs are just not worth it. Because when you reach my age you won't have anything to look back on, or have nothing to live off. You won't have education, you won't have a job, you won't have money, you will be constantly on job seekers allowance, and I know how much that is; that's £90 every two weeks and that's ridiculous.'

GANGS AND THE LAW

Although there are no laws banning gangs or gang membership, there are laws to prevent the criminal activity of gangs. These include:

- in court, if an offender was part of a gang, it could lead to a longer sentence
- drugs like cannabis, cocaine and ecstasy are illegal to have, or carry
- it is illegal to carry any knife if there is intent to use it as a weapon (even if it belongs to someone else)
- it is illegal to carry or keep a gun without a licence, including fake or replica guns
- police can search anyone they think may be carrying a gun or a knife
- police and school staff can also search young people for weapons at school.

Carrying a gun or a knife could mean being arrested, going to court and ending up with a criminal record that will affect the rest of that person's life. Having a criminal record can prevent people from getting a job, going to university or college, or even travelling abroad.

KNIVES AND THE LAW

What is and isn't legal

- It is illegal for any shop to sell a knife of any kind (including cutlery and kitchen knives) to anyone under the age of 18.
- It is an offence to carry a knife in public without good reason or lawful authority (for example, a chef on the way to work carrying his own knives has a good reason).
- The maximum penalty for an adult carrying a knife is four years in prison and a fine of £5 000.
- Knives where the blade folds into the handle, like a Swiss army knife, aren't illegal as long as the blade is shorter than three inches (7.62 centimetres).

Offensive weapons

If a knife is used in a threatening way (even a legal knife, such as a Swiss army knife), it is regarded as an 'offensive weapon' by the law. This is also the case with things like screwdrivers—once used in a threatening manner, they are treated as offensive weapons. It is an offence to carry an offensive weapon in a public place if you don't have a reasonable excuse. This means that carrying something that could be viewed as an offensive weapon, and then using it in a threatening way, could mean that you will be prosecuted. The penalty is up to four years' imprisonment and/or a fine.

There is a complete ban on the sale of certain types of knives categorised as offensive weapons, regardless of their use. These include:

- **flick knives**—Knives where the blade is hidden inside the handle and shoots out when a button is pressed; these are also called 'switchblades' or 'automatic knives'
- **butterfly knives**—Where the blade is hidden inside a handle that splits in two around it, like wings; the handles swing around the blade to open or close it
- **disguised knives**—Where the blade is hidden inside something like a belt buckle or fake mobile phone.

The police's 'stop and search' powers

Police officers have the right to search any person or vehicle if they suspect an offence—including carrying an offensive weapon.

Searches in schools and colleges

School staff in England have the power to search, without consent, any pupil they suspect of carrying a knife or other weapon in school or on an educational visit. Schools can also screen pupils at random, without suspicion, using a screening arch or an electronic 'wand'. Schools are not required by the law to inform a parent before performing a search, or to get parental consent. It is a criminal offence to bring a knife or other offensive weapon into school.[1]

 Invite the local police to come and present and field questions from the group.

SO HOW CAN WE HELP YOUNG PEOPLE AVOID BECOMING INVOLVED IN GANGS?

The challenge for adults is to create a framework that allows young people to discover who they are and what they believe in, to then be able to resist being influenced by the gang culture. There need to be opportunities for young people that:

- ensure they can see and be seen and feel valued
- ensure that they are part of a strong community
- help them develop a positive identity and have rites of passage that are understood by people they respect.

These are issues that can be supported by society as a whole. This would involve the statutory organisations within society such as the police and educational institutions as well as the family and community in general.[2]

- **The family and the community** are essential to the development of the child's social, emotional and physical needs. If the family is the source of love, guidance and protection that youths seek, they are not forced to search for these basic needs from a gang. Family and community share responsibility for teaching children the risk of drugs, etc., and give young people a sense of feeling valued, respected and heard.

- **Strong education and training** are directly related to a young person's positive development. Young people who successfully participate in and complete education have greater opportunities to develop into fulfilled adults. Adults can offer support and encouragement to see the value of education and to achieve. This does not necessarily need to be a traditional academic route but should also encompass apprenticeships and vocational routes.

- **Graffiti removal** reduces the chance that crimes will be committed. Since gangs use graffiti to mark their turf, advertise themselves, and claim credit for a crime, quick removal is essential.

- **Conflict resolution programmes** teach young people how to deal better with conflicts and help resist gang intimidation tactics.

- **Recreational programmes** such as sports, music, drama, and community activities help build a sense of self-worth and self-respect in young people. Young people involved in such activities are less likely to seek membership in a gang.

1 Invite professionals in to your organisation to speak and take questions on their job, how they got there, the satisfaction it brings, etc. You could invite a politician, lawyer, social worker or someone who is self employed. This gives a wider view of opportunities for the future and provides role models for the young people.

2 Invite creative groups to speak at your organization to raise awareness and inspire young people to become involved in what is happening in their local community. For instance, you could contact TA, Scouts, further education, vocational services, Connexions, etc.

3 Have an up-to-date notice board with what is going on for young people locally.

PROTECTIVE FACTORS

For individual young people there are protective factors that can help them to avoid joining gangs. These are some of the areas on which we can focus as professionals working with young people:

- well-developed social and interpersonal skills
- high sense of self-esteem, self-efficacy and personal responsibility
- reflectivity rather than impulsive thought and behavior
- internal locus of control (i.e. the belief that we are able to influence the environment in a positive manner)
- flexible coping strategies, well-developed problem-solving skills and intellectual abilities.

Self-esteem

The following are activities that can help young people become aware of how their self-esteem level affects their lives and will help them see the relationship between their self-esteem and the kinds of choices they make. They will also become aware of many of the things that they and other people do that either enhance or undermine their self-esteem, learn some ways to enhance their self-esteem, and become sensitized to the ways they affect the self-esteem of others.

Ranking traits

Ask the young people to rip a piece of paper into 10 strips. On each they should write a word or phrase that describes themselves.

Assure the young people that no one will see what they have written, so they can be extremely honest.

Ask each young person to arrange the traits in order from what he most likes about himself to what he likes least. Then ask him to give up one trait and ask how the lack of that trait affects him. Now give up another. Give up three. Then ask, 'Now what kind of person are you?' Give up six of these qualities in all. After giving up six of the qualities the young people can add back the traits one by one.

Explore with the young people any tension as they decide which traits they will give up. Discuss whether they feel incomplete without those traits. Explore whether they have a new understanding of the importance of those traits as they are regained.

Ask the young people to either share with the group or to write down what they learned about themselves from the experience.

Write yourself a letter

Ask the young people to write themselves a letter. Tell them that no one but them will read this letter, so they can say anything they want in it. However, a part of the letter might include who their friends are, their current height and weight, their favourite films and music, and special things both good and bad that occurred during the year. On another sheet of paper or the back of that sheet ask them to write 10 goals they would like to accomplish by this time next year. They then seal this letter in an envelope, self-address it, and give it to you. In a year, send the letters back to them.

This gives the young person the opportunity to set goals for the future, and on receipt of the letter to reflect on what they have achieved and where they have not achieved their goals. It also encourages them to explore why and to see where their goals have changed over the year.

Recognising talent and complementary talents

Begin by asking the young people, 'Who has something that they do really well?' After a brief discussion about some of those talents, pass out paper and ask them to write down five things that they do well.

Once they have all completed their list, ask for volunteers to share their lists.

Ask the young people to come up and select five different coloured paper strips. Using markers, ask them to write one talent on each strip of paper.

Demonstrate how to create a paper chain with their strips, linking their five talents together. As students begin to complete their mini chains, use extra strips of paper to link the mini chains together to create one long chain. Have students stand and hold the ever-growing chain as you link it together until all are linked.

Once the entire chain is constructed and linked together, and all the young people are standing holding each portion, ask them what this chain demonstrates. (This would be the fact that all the young people have talents that they do well.) Hang the chain up in the room as a reminder that the students are all good at something. Refer to it as needed during sessions with the young people.

Divide the group into pairs—ask the pairs to spend five to 10 minutes talking with each other. During their conversation, each person should find out his partner's name, age, something he has achieved in his lifetime, something he is good at and something he hopes to do in the future. They should then feed this back to the group. Giving voice to people's skills, achievements and goals improves self-esteem through language.

DEVELOPING PROBLEM-SOLVING SKILLS

There are plenty of formal and informal ways of developing problem-solving skills. A key principle in all these strategies is recognising that young people will do much better if they know they can solve their own problems, rather than having problems solved for them. This does not mean leaving them to sort these problems out alone: they benefit from adult support and confidence in learning ways of solving problems. But when adults offer advice and solutions too readily, this can frustrate the young person rather than help. The adult may also be irritated that their advice, offered with good intent, is not followed (they may often think to themselves that the young person just never listens or is just not motivated). It is better for both adult and young person that problems are explored, clarified and possibly redefined together before solutions suggested. Problem-solving requires the generation of both creative and critical thinking. It involves thinking about what is desired and what is possible.

And now for some games ...

Below are some game and activity suggestions here that can help people to see things differently and use different thinking styles. These games are stimulating, problem-solving tasks designed to help group members develop their capacity to work effectively together as well as hopefully being fun! You could make this a regular part of your group's activity.

Save the egg

Give the group an egg, two balloons, a roll of tape, some elastic bands, two straws and four pieces of paper.

The group has 20 minutes to make a vehicle to carry the egg. The vehicle should be strong enough to withstand a small drop onto concrete.

Community quest

This is a great activity for building teamwork, learning about the services available in your community and updating your resource files.

Divide the group into teams of four to eight. Each team should include young people and adults. Each team receives a list of items for a scavenger hunt for information about community services. *Examples:* a brochure from a runaway shelter; a brochure from the teen health centre, etc.

Teams are given a deadline to return for a pizza/ice cream/ whatever you like party. The team with the most items wins a small prize. Your community and the interests of your group will determine the items on the list.

Flip the rug

Give the group a small rug or a sheet big enough for them to stand on comfortably. Ask them to stand on the rug. They must flip the rug over with out stepping off it.

Paper folding

You will need several sheets of large paper (size A2). Chairs and tables should be available around the room but should not be pointed out to the young people.

Split the young people into groups of four or five. Place a piece of paper in front of each group and tell them they have five seconds to get off the floor. The group will automatically jump onto the paper. Then tell the groups that you want them to fold the paper in half and they then have another five seconds to get off the floor ... repeat this until they have folded the paper 6 or more times. The idea of the game is that the young people will automatically fold the paper and stand on it using each other as supports when all they actually had to do was fold the paper as instructed, then get off the floor—they could have sat on a chair or table in the room!

SYSTEMATIC PROBLEM-SOLVING

Young people who have a sense of loss of personal control may turn to peer groups that foster hate and lash out at those individuals who are perceived to be different. Those who are adept at positive social interactions feel more in control of their lives, decreasing their need to join radical fringe groups that promote crime and racial intolerance. Those who are disliked by others do not form bonds with others. Not having satisfying friendships, they often turn to antisocial behaviour, seeking activities that are stimulating to them. Young people without friends often resort to alcohol and drug use and engage in gang behavior. Those who do not have a wide range of positive social skills to draw from to deal with stress become disconnected from positive values, high standards for one's behavior and responsibility. They feel alienated from the higher concepts of respect for others and democracy.

The games are a fun way of problem solving, drawing on the strengths of those in the group to work together. Out in the real world the young people may have problems they would like to examine to learn how they can deal with them in a constructive manner. The following process can be helpful in supporting them in this. You could do this as a group activity with some hypothetical scenarios; and if you feel confident and a young person approaches you with a specific situation you can support him or her through this process individually. For the latter it is vital to stay impartial, help the young person to see the options available, stay within the boundaries of law, and be aware of confidentiality issues. It is always worth discussing this with a colleague to ensure that you are supported.

This approach, which is particularly useful for dealing with social and learning-based problems, involves the following six steps:

1. Defining the problem

The aim is to get a shared agreement on what exactly the problem is. Often there are different perspectives to a problem. A teacher might have a problem if a student has not done his homework. The student might have the problem that he or she doesn't have somewhere to do his homework. If there is shared definition that the difficulty is, say, how the child can find somewhere to do the work, then the process of finding a solution can begin.

2. Generating ideas

This is the process of thinking about all the things that might possibly be done to solve the problem. It is important to accept all ideas suggested. Often, children may be reluctant to offer ideas for fear they will be criticised as impractical or dismissed. Writing everything down sends a strong message that they are being taken seriously. If the young person who can't find a place to do his homework suggests that he doesn't do it, write this suggestion down, but invite him to keep thinking of other strategies.

3. Critically evaluating ideas

Once a list has been generated that contains some feasible ideas, then it is time to think some of them through. Sometimes, ideas can be grouped together. To help evaluate them, it can be useful to ask questions that link actions with consequences. For instance, 'If you do that, what would happen next?' or 'How would others respond?' From all these ideas, select the ones worth trying and discard those not worth pursuing or that no one wants to discuss.

4. Selecting a solution

From the possibilities generated, select one to try. If necessary, develop an action plan. The child needs to have commitment to try it out, so the more he or she is involved in the selection process and the final choice, the better. It is important that any solution fits with the organisation's values and beliefs about what is acceptable behaviour.

5. Trying it out

6. Evaluating the solution

Arrange a follow-up where you can hear about what has happened and whether the problem has been resolved. If it has, give positive feedback.

You could start by asking for suggestions of problems to be solved from the group so the process could be modeled with them. Alternatively there may be problems that arise during your work with the young people and this process will help work through to arrive at socially acceptable solutions.

Working with Gangs and Young People: a toolkit for resolving group conflict

By Jessie Feinstein and Nia Imani Kuumba
www.youthwork.com/activitiesinit.html

Additional resources

This valuable website is dedicated to combating knife crime:
www.bebo.com/itdoesnthavetohappen

REFERENCES

1. www.direct.gov.uk/en/CrimeJusticeAndTheLaw/index.htm
2. www.focusas.com/Gangs.html

Glossary

Aluminium chloride: A compound of aluminium and chlorine. Forms a plug in sweat ducts and kills bacteria.

Aluminium zirconium: Plugs sweat glands and absorbs moisture.

Anabolic steroids: Drugs which mimic the effects of the male sex hormones testosterone and dihydrotestosterone. They increase protein synthesis within cells, which results in the buildup of cellular tissue (anabolism), especially in muscles. Anabolic steroids also have androgenic and virilizing properties, including the development and maintenance of masculine characteristics such as the growth of the vocal cords and body hair.

Anaemia: A decrease in number of red blood cells or less than the normal quantity of hemoglobin in the blood.

Anorexia: Being underweight.

Anorexia nervosa: An eating disorder characterized by refusal to maintain a healthy body weight and an obsessive fear of gaining weight, often coupled with a distorted self-image.

Autistic spectrum: A spectrum of psychological conditions characterized by abnormalities of social interactions and communication, as well as restricted interests and repetitive behaviour.

Bacteria: One-celled organisms; various species of which are involved in fermentation, putrefaction, infectious diseases or nitrogen fixation.

Bipolar disorder: An affective disorder characterized by periods of mania alternating with periods of depression, usually interspersed with relatively long intervals of normal mood.

Cardiovascular: Of the heart and blood vessels.

Chronic heart failure: Inability of the heart to supply sufficient blood flow to meet the body's needs.

Crohn's disease: A chronic inflammatory bowel disease that causes scarring and thickening of the intestinal walls and frequently leads to obstruction.

Cystic fibrosis: A hereditary, chronic disease of the exocrine glands, characterized by the production of mucus that obstructs the pancreatic ducts and bronchi, leading to infection and fibrosis.

Dental dam:
1 Also called 'rubber dam'; a thin piece of latex placed over the tooth or teeth being treated during dental work.
2 A thin piece of latex used to prevent the transfer of bodily fluids during cunnilingus or anilingus.

Depilatory: Capable of removing hair.

Depressant: Having the quality of depressing or lowering the vital activities; sedative.

Diabetes: A disorder of carbohydrate metabolism characterized by inadequate production or use of insulin and resulting in excessive amounts of glucose in the blood and urine, excessive thirst, weight loss, and in some cases progressive destruction of small blood vessels leading to complications such as infections and gangrene of the limbs or blindness.

Ectopic pregnancy: The development of a fertilized ovum outside the uterus, as in a uterine tube.

Electrolyte: Any of certain inorganic compounds, mainly sodium, potassium, magnesium, calcium, chloride, and bicarbonate, that dissociate in biological fluids into ions capable of conducting electrical currents and constituting a major force in controlling fluid balance within the body.

Emphysema: A chronic, irreversible disease of the lungs characterized by abnormal enlargement of air spaces in the lungs accompanied by destruction of the tissue lining the walls of the air spaces.

Epidemiology: The science dealing with the incidence and prevalence of disease in large populations and with detection of the source and cause of epidemics of infectious disease.

Epilepsy: A disorder of the nervous system, characterized either by mild, episodic loss of attention or sleepiness (petit mal) or by severe convulsions with loss of consciousness (grand mal).

Folate: Any of a group of vitamins of the B complex; from Latin *folium* leaf, because it may be obtained from green leaves.

Fungi: Any of a diverse group of eukaryotic single-celled or multinucleate organisms that live by decomposing and absorbing the organic material in which they grow, comprising the mushrooms, moulds, mildews, smuts, rusts and yeasts, and classified in the kingdom Fungi.

Gestation: The period of time spent in the uterus between conception and birth.

Glaucoma: Abnormally high fluid pressure in the eye.

Haemoglobin: A conjugated protein, consisting of haem and the protein globin, that gives red blood cells their characteristic colour. It combines reversibly with oxygen and is thus very important in the transportation of oxygen to tissues.

Hallucinations: A sensory experience of something that does not exist outside the mind, caused by various physical and mental disorders, or by reaction to certain toxic substances, and usually manifested as visual or auditory images.

Heart disease: Any condition of the heart that impairs its functioning.

Hepatitis: Inflammation of the liver, caused by a virus or a toxin and characterized by jaundice, liver enlargement, and fever.

Hypothalamus: A region of the brain, between the thalamus and the midbrain, that functions as the main control centre for the autonomic nervous system by regulating sleep cycles, body temperature, appetite, etc., and that acts as an endocrine gland by producing hormones, including the releasing factors that control the hormonal secretions of the pituitary gland.

Iron deficiency anaemia: A form of anaemia due to lack of iron in the diet or to iron loss as a result of chronic bleeding.

Latex: A milky liquid in certain plants that coagulates on exposure to air.

Laxative: A medicine or agent for relieving constipation.

Libido: Sexual instinct or sexual drive.

Lipoprotein: Any of a group of proteins to which a lipid molecule is attached, important in the transport of lipids in the bloodstream.

Liver cirrhosis: A disease of the liver characterised by increase in connective tissue and alteration in gross and microscopic makeup.

Makaton: A language that uses signs, symbols and speech to help people with learning and/or communication difficulties to communicate.

Manic: A type of affective disorder characterized by euphoric mood, excessive activity and talkativeness, impaired judgment and sometimes psychotic symptoms, as grandiose delusions.

Manic depression: A mental health problem characterized by an alternation between extreme euphoria and deep depression.

Neurotoxin: Poisonous to the nerves.

Noxious: Harmful or injurious to health or physical well-being.

Obsessive compulsive disorder: A common mental health problem. Symptoms typically include recurring obsessive thoughts, and repetitive compulsions in response to the obsession.

Osteoporosis: A disorder in which the bones become increasingly porous, brittle and subject to fracture due to loss of calcium and other mineral components, sometimes resulting in pain, decreased height and skeletal deformities: common in older persons, primarily postmenopausal women, but also associated with long-term steroid therapy and certain endocrine disorders.

Pelvic: Of the pelvis.

Pelvic inflammatory disease: An inflammation of the female pelvic organs, most commonly the uterine tubes, usually as a result of bacterial infection.

Pituitary gland: A small, cherry-shaped double structure attached by a stalk to the base of the brain and constituting the master endocrine gland affecting all hormonal functions in the body.

Podophylin: A resin, occurring as a light brown to greenish amorphous powder, obtained from podophyllum, and used in medicine chiefly as a purgative and, locally, in the treatment of genital warts.

Podophyllum gets its name from the Greek words *podos* and *phyllon*, meaning foot-shaped leaves. Podophyllum rhizomes have a long medicinal history among native North American tribes who used a rhizome powder as a laxative or an agent that expels worms (anthelmintic). A poultice of the powder was also used to treat warts and tumorous growths on the skin.

Polyurethane: A thermoplastic polymer. A thermoplastic is a polymer that turns to a liquid when heated and freezes to a very glassy state when cooled. A polymer is a large molecule (macromolecule) composed of repeating structural units. These subunits are typically connected by covalent chemical bonds.

Prostate gland: An organ that surrounds the urethra of males at the base of the bladder and comprising a muscular portion, which controls the release of urine, and a glandular portion, which secretes an alkaline fluid that makes up part of the semen and enhances the motility and fertility of sperm.

Psychomotor: Of or pertaining to a response involving both motor and psychological components.

Psychosis: A mental disorder characterized by symptoms, such as delusions or hallucinations, that indicate impaired contact with reality.

Schizophrenia: A severe mental disorder characterized by some, but not necessarily all, of the following features: emotional blunting, intellectual deterioration, social isolation, disorganized speech and behaviour, delusions and hallucinations.

Steroids: Any of a large group of fat-soluble organic compounds, as the sterols, bile acids, and sex hormones, most of which have specific physiological action.

Stimulant: Something that temporarily quickens some vital process or the functional activity of some organ or part.

Stroke: A blockage or haemorrhage of a blood vessel leading to the brain, causing inadequate oxygen supply and, depending on the extent and location of the abnormality, weakness, paralysis of parts of the body, speech difficulties, and if severe, loss of consciousness or death.

Synthetic: Man-made.

Tourette's syndrome: A neurological disorder characterized by recurrent involuntary movements, including multiple neck jerks and sometimes vocal tics as grunts, barks or words, especially obscenities.

Ultrasound:
1 Physics: Sound with a frequency greater than 20 000 Hz, approximately the upper limit of human hearing.
2 Medicine/medical: The application of ultrasonic waves to therapy or diagnostics, as in deep-heat treatment of a joint or imaging of internal structures.

Vascular: Pertaining to, composed of, or provided with vessels or ducts that convey fluids, as blood, lymph or sap.

Vasodilation: The widening of blood vessels resulting from relaxation of smooth muscle cells within the vessel walls, particularly in the large arteries, smaller arterioles and large veins.

Vegan: A vegetarian who omits all animal products from the diet.

Ventricular: Of the ventricle: A chamber of the heart that receives blood from one or more atria and pumps it by muscular contraction into the arteries.

Virus: An ultramicroscopic (20 to 300 nm in diameter), metabolically inert, infectious agent that replicates only within the cells of living hosts, mainly bacteria, plants and animals: composed of an RNA or DNA core, a protein coat, and in more complex types, a surrounding envelope.

Index

Figures and diagrams are given in italics